PENGUIN BOOKS

THE BRINK OF BEING

Julia Bueno is a psychotherapist who specializes in working with women who have experienced pregnancy loss or struggled to conceive. Her writing has been published in *The Times* (London), *Express*, *Therapy Today*, and welldoing .org, among others. She lives in London with her husband and two sons.

The Brink of Being

TALKING ABOUT MISCARRIAGE

Julia Bueno

PENGUIN BOOKS

PENGUIN BOOKS
An imprint of Penguin Random House LLC
penguinrandomhouse.com

First published in Great Britain by Virago Press 2019
Published in Penguin Books 2019

LIBRARY OF CONGRESS CATALOGING-IN-PUBLICATION DATA

Names: Bueno, Julia, author.
Title: The brink of being : talking about miscarriage / Julia Bueno.
Description: New York : Penguin Books, [2019] | Includes
bibliographical references and index.
Identifiers: LCCN 2019000494 (print) | LCCN 2019000577 (ebook) |
ISBN 9780525505013 (ebook) | ISBN 9780143133230 (paperback)
Subjects: LCSH: Miscarriage. | Miscarriage--Psychological aspects.
Classification: LCC RG648 (ebook) | LCC RG648 .B84 2019 (print) |
DDC 618.3/92--dc23
LC record available at https://lccn.loc.gov/2019000494

ISBN 9780143133230 (paperback)
ISBN 9780525505013 (ebook)

Printed in the United States of America
1 3 5 7 9 10 8 6 4 2

DESIGNED BY AMANDA DEWEY

For David

Contents

Introduction

It is commonly estimated that one in four pregnancies fails to thrive, and ends spontaneously in a miscarriage—most before they have been revealed to the world, or even suggested by the hint of a pregnancy bump. This can be devastating, extremely physically painful, or both. And yet despite its prevalence, we have been long unable to talk about miscarriage in any adequate breadth or depth. If we do, we tend to do so awkwardly, quickly, and in the most general terms. We squirm, we whisper, and we avoid asking questions— we just don't understand the experience well enough or the nature of the complex grief that can hit hard in its wake.

But miscarriage deserves so much more than these scant responses it tends to elicit. We need to approach this human experience with greater empathy and an allied compassionate curiosity so that, ultimately, we can improve the support that's on offer for all of those who may be affected. I began to learn this in the wake of my own miscarriages: my first one profoundly changed me, inspired a new career, and still fuels my desire to change how miscarriage is perceived.

The inklings of my future family began when I was eighteen years old and met my now husband, David, on my first day of college. He and his friend had spotted me walking through the swing door of a building near their rooms, on my way to visit a friend. I later found them both lying on the ground, blocking my exit. I laughed, we all talked, and then the friend peeled off, leaving David and me to talk some more. Later that night David introduced me to Van Morrison, and by the time I returned to my room, I knew that I wanted to spend the rest of my life with him. It took another year before he agreed.

We both wanted children, but parenthood wasn't on the agenda for a long time. While David fell into journalism soon after graduating, I flirted with academia and then a legal career, before moving to an internet start-up. But after a decade together, we had bought our first home in London and were planning a wedding. Having a baby seemed like the next step, and as soon as David agreed to try, a baby was all I wanted. And I wanted it to be like the story I knew the best: I'd get pregnant before too long, grow fat and uncomfortable, and then give birth to a little version of him and me.

But this story would never be told. For us, things took a different turn from the beginning. I had spent many years ignoring my irregular menstrual cycle, disguising what I suspected was a minor fertility issue with the synthetic hormones of the contraceptive pill. When we first discussed trying to conceive, we consulted my sensible general practitioner, who sent me for further investigations. I assumed if anything was awry, there would be a simple fix.

After a scan revealed some unusual findings, I was sent for a laparoscopy—a tiny fiber-optic cable was inserted through my abdomen wall to inspect the state of my womb and ovaries. An hour or so later, as I awoke from my drugged sleep of general anesthesia in the recovery ward, my surgeon appeared, his wild white hair only partly tamed by a surgeon's cap. He excitedly reported what the camera had revealed: I have a unicornuate uterus—a malformation that means my uterus didn't fully develop when I was in my mother's womb. It is, in keeping with the medical inclination to describe wombs as varieties of fruit, shaped like a banana, rather than the avocado Mother Nature prefers.

My surgeon also told me that while I had two functioning ovaries, I now had only one fallopian tube; the other was barely developed and useless, so he had removed it during the procedure. He handed it to me in a small plastic jar: a gray gnarled lump of flesh. Baffled at my gift, I was also soothed by the promise of a healthy counterpart. At a follow-up appointment a month later, he was upbeat about my prognosis to conceive and carry a baby to term. My anomalies may have explained my irregular menstrual cycle, and he glossed over the increased risk of pregnancy loss or premature delivery that my abnormal womb could potentially cause. He told me gripping stories of other strange-shaped wombs that had resulted in happy deliveries. I left his consulting room buoyant and with a renewed sense of expectation: an experienced doctor thought a pregnancy could, and would, happen for me.

It took about a year of hopes raised and then dashed before I conceived. I was so consumed with my desire to get pregnant that it eclipsed everything else, including our wedding. I didn't care about the details of my dress or which flowers to choose as much as the repeated arrival of my period. But, at long last, a couple of months before my thirtieth birthday and ten months after our wedding, my familiar bleeding didn't arrive, and I took my first pregnancy test. I still have the white plastic wand that proved I had conceived the baby (and, it turned out, another baby) that had long been nestled in my mind.

It was only a couple of weeks after my pregnancy was confirmed that our joy was punctured by fears. First, I started to spot—a common experience of light bleeding in early pregnancy that can be caused by the embryo implanting itself in the womb lining. A scan at the hospital at around six weeks revealed this was probably the case with me, but it also revealed two minuscule humans with beating hearts: I had conceived twins. Growing two babies inside a banana-shaped womb within my five-foot frame was never going to be easy, but I remembered the words of my surgeon. And I hoped.

The coming weeks brought even more anxiety: I had bouts of sudden and heavy bleeding. More scans showed that a sizable hemorrhage had formed in my womb lining and was struggling to heal. I was told that this was probably because my womb had stretched too rapidly—not unheard of with first pregnancies of twins. I became a frequent flyer of the high-risk pregnancy unit, led by an obstetrician with legendary expertise in twin pregnancies. I bled copiously, and often, throughout the following ten weeks, while also battling intense and relentless nausea that made it difficult to eat. And while our frequent hospital visits assured us that our babies were thriving nonetheless, there were few moments during my first trimester when I could relax into my dreams of a future family of four.

But then at around sixteen weeks, during yet another checkup, a scan showed that the familiar dark patch on my womb lining had disappeared. Suddenly and inexplicably, the hemorrhage had healed. Our hope renewed, I contacted a local support group for new mothers of multiples, and my husband and I began to work out how we would share childcare. My mother started amassing a collection of tiny clothes, and my belly expanded so much that people leaped up from their seats on buses to offer me theirs. We played with names and flew to Italy for a friend's wedding, where I danced all night in a dress that I bought a few sizes too big.

This excitement lasted only a month. One sweltering summer's day twenty weeks into the pregnancy, before leaving for work, I went to the loo and, habituated to check the bowl for blood, I spotted something new. I didn't see a pool of deep red, but a dark green blob of flesh-like tissue. I had read enough to know that this was my mucus plug—the seal that forms at the neck of the womb to keep infection out. I also knew it could mean that labor would come soon. I called my office to say I would be late—again—and walked to my nearby doctor, eating an unripe nectarine and clinging to an absurd hope that she would assure me that my body was already busy making a replacement mucus plug. But deep down I think I knew the truth: that my pregnancy was under serious threat.

Without even examining me, the doctor fast-tracked me to the hospital unit that David and I already knew so well. David met me there, as dazed as I was. A scan showed that my cervix was giving way, which would have been fine if it were October, rather than July, halfway through my second trimester. My straight-talking obstetrician swiftly made a decision to stitch it, or, as he said, what was left of it. I had gotten to know his curious bedside manner well over the previous weeks under his care—it was a small trade for his dedication to guarding the safety of complex twin pregnancies. There was no time to go through the usual preoperative rigmarole of fasting, and I was rushed to surgery that night.

I awoke in the twilight hours of the following morning, itchy from the morphine, with a nurse filling in my chart beside a small lamp in the room. My mind organized itself slowly, registering relief to feel limbs still moving inside me. The nurse and I talked about the chickens she kept and her constant fear of foxes. I learned that she had had many miscarriages, never fulfilling her dream to be a mother. Her hope for my babies to remain safe inside me for as long as possible was palpable. She held my hand as I fell asleep, and I didn't see her again.

By the time my cervix was stitched that night, we had already grown familiar with the exquisitely formed tiny features of each of our babies, revealed in grainy black and white during my frequent scans. A tiny version of my husband's nose emerged on one girl, and the other baby vacillated between being my son or my daughter, depending on its position. I had become used to the discomfort of eight limbs moving around inside of me, along with the strangest of shapes being made out of my belly when I lay down. I had never looked so big or felt so amazed at what my body had made, and become.

On his morning round, my obstetrician assured David and me that he had done his best to keep my womb closed. He couldn't tell me if his stitch would hold—"it will be what it will be," he said, or something along those lines. And while we were desperate to know of the odds for two live— and healthy—births, all he could do was to send me home to "take it easy," although I was to avoid bed rest and, essentially, to cross my fingers. As I went on to learn, as with so many aspects of miscarriage, there are frustratingly stunted amounts of helpful knowledge.

If I made it to twenty-eight weeks—another two months—there would be a good chance of my babies both surviving, and thriving, without lasting health problems. Advances in neonatal care mean that the viability of babies born too early has grown hugely over recent years, but my babies had no chance of surviving on their own if they had been born when my stitch was put in. We all knew that the longer I could stay pregnant, the better. So, fearful of a stress- ful commute threatening my pregnancy, I set up an office at home and began my crawl through the treacle of time. Each day that passed felt like a mini-victory, yet however much I tried not to, I was also bracing myself for the worst.

Two weeks into my self-enforced confinement, in the twenty-second week of pregnancy, I awoke in excruciating pain. It felt as if a bolt of searing metal had been forced through my lower back and into my pelvis. I woke David with the words we had both been dreading: "I'm in labor." Desperate to get me to the hospital quickly, he bundled me into our car. All I remember of the journey is resting my weight on four limbs on the backseat, vomiting through each wave of pain into a filthy plastic bag—the only thing we could find. When I opened my eyes between what I assumed were contractions, I saw flashes of white.

With David supporting me, I stumbled into the hospital's labor ward, and a small ocean of straw-colored water gushed out of me, onto the floor by the reception desk. David had called in advance, so they were expecting me. A soft-spoken midwife ushered us into a room. She told me she was deaf and relied on lipreading. Determined not to offend her, I waited for her back to turn to scream and swear. I can still see her face, pushed up close to mine as she translated my lip movements into repeated requests for pain relief.

Doctors came and went. Midwives came and went. Eventually it emerged that they were holding back from appeasing my requests for pain relief while they worked out if it was possible to stop the course of labor. But while the medics dithered, I knew that I couldn't keep my babies safe: my body was doing what it was clearly determined to do. My cervix had opened, and its stitch of promise was lost in the cleaned-away mess of amniotic fluid on the floor. Eventually, everyone agreed: my babies would be born, and they were too young to survive. I will never know exactly when it was that their hearts stopped beating.

An epidural was put into my lower back and the pain

from the throes of contractions ebbed away. Labor then slowed down, and my gentle midwife finished her shift. She was replaced with Mat, who took my hands and looked me in the eye before he did anything else. I remain deeply grateful to whoever drew up the rotation for that week on that ward: he got me through the hours of living hell that followed. He knew far better than I what my womb was doing and how labor worked, and he was tireless in his desire to ease my emotional and physical pain. He also understood why I repeatedly begged—screamed—for a cesarean section. I did not want to push two dying, or dead, babies out of me.

At some point later on, an obviously harassed young obstetrician appeared at my side with a deadpan face and air of irritation. "If I perform a C-section on you," he told me bluntly, "I risk rupturing your womb and you'll never have a baby again. So, have another think about it." He left as abruptly as he had arrived, and Mat translated his stinging words into kinder ones that I was better able to understand.

Matilda was born a couple of hours after that, with David by my side. She delivered herself, weighing a whisper over a pound, with Mat receiving her. I fell asleep. Three, four, six hours later—I still don't know, but it was the next day, and the first day of the next month—her sister, Florence, was born weighing just under a pound. I had to push this time, with Mat instructing me how to and when, as I knew nothing about giving birth. Nothing I had read about pregnancy prepared me for such an event. He took her to join her sister, who had already been placed somewhere else, by I don't know who, in another universe.

I remember feeling relief that it was all over. I think I made a quip about how hungry I was, and asked David to go and buy me my favorite sandwich from a nearby shop. I couldn't bear to think about what had just happened. My mother and my sister appeared by my side soon after that, as more blood was taken from my veins and my epidural and cannula were removed. They met Mat, before he left for home, hours after his shift had officially ended. Nine months later, back at the same hospital with a newly born, very premature son, I tried to find him, but he had moved on.

Another midwife tried to persuade David and me to meet our daughters before they were taken to the hospital mortuary for their postmortem that she had hurriedly, uncomfortably, discussed with us. I didn't want to see them. I also did want to see them, but I was too shocked, too frightened, and too disbelieving. I wanted to hold on to memories of my babies when they had been alive, kicking inside me, and so did David. Eventually, she heard our wishes, but I live with the deep regret that she didn't give me more time for my shock to settle. My mother and sister did want to meet their new family members, and we agreed to let them be the keepers of their earthly existence.

I was taken to a bathroom opposite the delivery room. Alone, I washed the births away in a bubble bath while I listened to the wails of a baby in the next room and the screams of a laboring mother in another. Having just delivered babies too, I felt a warm trace of kinship with this other mother, but I couldn't bear to hear the other tiny cries. I dried off and put on the stained pajamas in which I had arrived. A midwife handed me a clear plastic bag with painkillers, folded papers, two white cards with a pair of pink footprints on each, and two polaroid photographs—the only tangible evidence I would have of my babies' births and deaths.

I then stepped back out into the world as a woman who had just had a miscarriage. This was a world that would struggle to understand both the physical process that I had been through and the agonizing nature of my everlasting grief. A world that didn't want to know the details of what had happened, let alone remember them; a world that didn't know if I was a mother or David a father or whether my two babies had been born or whether they had actually died. This world was poorly equipped to support me—and the countless other women and couples I soon discovered who were also reeling in their own versions of such pain.

"MISCARRIAGE" REFERS TO the most common complication of early pregnancy and is often quoted to affect one in four pregnancies. If you or your partner hasn't suffered one, you will know someone who has—even though you may not even know it. One estimate suggests that in the USA, 750,000 to 1,000,000 pregnancies end this way each year, yet a recent US national survey found that it was popularly believed to be an uncommon complication. Another estimate for the UK suggested that 684 miscarriages happened each day in 2016. It is most likely to happen in the first twelve weeks of pregnancy, although it can also happen well after the first trimester too—up until the time it is legally deemed a stillbirth. In the UK, this means up until the twenty-fourth week of pregnancy, while in the US and Australia this boundary lies a month earlier.

Since research papers refer only to miscarriages in pregnancies that have been diagnosed medically, and not to those diagnosed at home with a shop-bought pregnancy test, it's possible that our estimates are low. Also, given that a greater proportion of women are choosing to delay childbearing and the risk of miscarriage increases with maternal age, miscarriage rates may be increasing. A report from the Office for National Statistics for England and Wales in 2015 found that women aged forty and over had a higher fertility rate (i.e., incidence of live births) than women under twenty, a disparity last recorded in the wake of World War II. This trend is reflected in other countries in Western Europe, Australia, New Zealand, Canada, and the USA.

But the prevalence of miscarriage bears no relation to how it is talked about and understood. If anything, it may have contributed to its relegation to a "mere" risk of reproduction that can happen to the best of us. But my first miscarriage rapidly taught me how disastrous other misperceptions could be to the passage of my grief: my adult life now hinges around this event, and I subsequently discovered how many other people also felt their miscarriages scored similarly deeply into their life—and family—narrative.

There is the "before," and there is the "after." When Matilda and Florence died, other parts of me did too. I left the hospital that day knowing that I couldn't count on my body to make a baby who would live to be my child, but also as someone who was fundamentally different from the person I was before. My confidence and self-worth plummeted to unprecedented depths. And as the following weeks blurred into one another, this lack of faith in myself trickled out to most people around me, who I came to believe would also let me down. My anger, bitterness, and sadness could be so acute at times that my chest would burn—and I was a difficult person to be around. I was quick to anger, quick to judge, and frequently sarcastic. I understand this now to be a price of love, and of a broken heart, but it was far more than that too.

A lack of adequate understanding and support for the complexity of what had happened to me contributed to my despair. Very few people around me took the time to find out the details of what had happened before, during, and after my miscarriage, and I felt intense pressure to move on and get pregnant again. I felt desperately, painfully alone. But I did move on, conceiving my now sixteen-year-old son just three months after we left the hospital empty-armed. This made for a pregnancy steeped in guilt and high anxiety, and my grief struggled to find the space it really needed. I still wonder how much of my motivation to conceive so quickly came from a desire to distract myself, as well as others, from the unbearable incompatibility between birth and death that my first pregnancy had brought about.

After the birth of my son, I went on to have three more miscarriages, which were made so much worse by things said—and not said—to me. We bereaved tend to remember these things well. With notable exceptions, many people around me got it, unwittingly, wrong each time. I was repeatedly told that "at least" these miscarriages were earlier on, and my hospital experiences could be easily subsumed into the medical events they became, along with their admission and discharge notes. Thinly spread compassion waned as my unlucky reproductive story continued: my fourth miscarriage was barely acknowledged at all by friends, colleagues, or family, and it even seemed to irritate those keen for me to get over my seemingly deranged desire to have another baby.

It's not that these people are mean or uncaring. Some of them were overworked and underpaid yet dedicated medical staff who weren't adequately trained to deal with miscarriage; others were friends in the grip of an outdated, unchallenged cultural rule to not mention it. Maybe some were squeamish and wanted to avoid the thought of blood, clots, tissues, pain, and embryonic bodies. After all, periods, prolapses, birth traumas, breast milk, menopauses, and other aspects of women's health are also topics of whispered and uneasy conversations, if not disgust. I also know that others thought it best not to stir my splintery upset by talking about the *m* word.

But there were also others who genuinely wondered, out of ignorance rather than malice, what all the fuss was about. I hadn't ever lost a child who had breathed on earth: confusion prevails where an experience is so immersed in ambiguity and riddled with paradox. Miscarriage tussles with "sort ofs" and "almosts" and "if onlys," teetering in between life and death, parenthood and childlessness, the public and private realms, mental and physical health. It seemed strenuous for people to accept the enormity of both the real and potential loss a miscarriage can bring. It's no wonder I lacked enough support, when we can't yet wrap our heads around these conflicts and indefinable ideas.

My experiences—both of the bad and the exceptionally supportive few—inspired me to train as a telephone support volunteer for the UK's leading charity dedicated to miscarriage, the Miscarriage Association. I had learned the value of talking to someone who was prepared to listen and be genuinely curious and understanding about my experiences, and I wanted to offer the same. Despite the Miscarriage Association's continuing influence on miscarriage care, health policies, and the support of the bereaved, it remains a relatively tiny charity, compared with others devoted to babies lost later in gestation or at full-term birth. I later became a trustee and worked hard with the board to raise awareness and promote the understanding of what miscarriage can involve—both within and outside of hospital walls.

Over a decade later, while both miscarriage care in medical settings and cultural understanding have improved greatly, the charity's work is far from done, and research edges only incrementally toward a better understanding of what prevents pregnancies from thriving to their rightful end. My work with the Miscarriage Association and the talking therapy that I turned to in my loneliness and grief lay behind my decision to retrain as a psychotherapist. After fifteen years in consulting rooms in various public and private services, I have talked to hundreds of women—and some partners—about their miscarriages. While I am heartened by the positive changes in medical care and cultural understanding that have been made since I started my work,

I also know we still have a long way to go before the anguish of those who have undergone a miscarriage earns settled coordinates on the map of grief.

IN THIS BOOK, I explore experiences of miscarriage and their broader cultural, medical, and historical context in rarely heard intimate detail. I want to bring you up close to the physical and emotional tolls that can be endured in early, late, and repeated miscarriage, along with the medical interventions and decision making that may be necessary at such vulnerable times—including the agonizing considerations of what we do with a miscarried baby's body and the breast milk it was destined to suckle.

I want you—whether you have been affected by miscarriage or simply desire to learn more about it—to think further about how we define pregnancies, birth, death, parenthood, and grief, as well as the tensions that arise when medicine rubs up against the emotional, intuitive realm of human grief and loss. Although each chapter is discrete, the themes and ideas within them overlap and echo across the book: what applies to an early loss may well apply to a loss at a later gestation, and what applies to the experience of repeated miscarriage may well apply to the experience of having only one. Having said that, I think the chapters are best read in sequence.

In the first chapter, I explore the potentially profound relationship that can come into being with a barely conceived or even unconceived baby, which lays the foundations for profound grief when a pregnancy ends. We know that most miscarriages happen early on in pregnancy—before twelve weeks—and the second chapter concentrates on some of the particularities of such early loss. In the rarer case of late miscarriage, which I explore next, people may be more willing to accept the existence of a "baby" and "birth" and "death" than with miscarriages of earlier gestations, but these still remain precarious notions, and the details of hospital experiences are often not known outside of hospital walls. I then go on to explore the grueling nature of repeated miscarriage—a rarer, but by no means statistically insignificant, experience that requires another realm of emotional endurance. My penultimate chapter considers the impact of miscarriage on partners and other family members. I close with a look at what is probably the least familiar aspect of miscarriage: how we choose to dispose of, and remember, the family member who never made it to the family tree.

The clients I write about are composite people, based on the hundreds of stories I have listened to, and not always in a consulting room: I have heard stories about miscarriage while walking on beaches and along corridors, on trains and coaches, and even at weddings and baptisms. I have also read blogs, memoirs, and threads from support groups, in addition to attending face-to-face groups. I have not divulged any information in breach of client confidentiality, and I have ensured that individuals are unidentifiable, where appropriate. That is not to say that some people may think they recognize themselves in some of the circumstances I have described as there may well be coincidences and commonalities. Some details have been included with an explicit request to do so, as a gift for the book's campaign: to enlighten as many people as possible about an experience that is clothed by so much misunderstanding.

While I use stories from my consulting room, I write almost nothing about the therapeutic process. The art and skill of psychotherapy after miscarriage is a worthy subject for another book, but that is not my focus here. I have also almost always kept the fact of my own miscarriages hidden from my clients, for fear of intruding on their stories. I thought long and hard about revealing some of the most intimate details of my life here, and took a risk in the belief that—like the other stories I recount—they will be of help to those who can recognize them or of interest to those who want to learn more. These memories of mine are inevitably subject to some inaccuracies that the passage of time, and layers of powerful feelings, have unwittingly created.

I can't possibly describe every experience of losing a baby too soon, and some of the parameters that I have drawn may seem arbitrary to some readers. The experience of miscarriage skirts as closely to that of a stillbirth as possible, as well as to the potential agony, or relief, of an elective termination made for medical or other reasons. Rather than widening my lens in what might be appropriate and obvious ways, I have chosen to do justice, as best I can, to the experience of pregnancy loss that I know about the most.

There is a lamentable lack of research into the experience of miscarriage among many cultural and religious groups—as well as that of male partners, same-sex couples, teenagers, and women and couples with learning disabilities. But as with all other aspects of research into this field, I am hopeful that these essential changes are beginning to happen, partly with the help of current anthropological research. While I am confident that my stories faithfully draw on the experiences of a significant number of people, I also acknowledge that they represent only a small number of the bereaved after miscarriage—the secular, and English-speaking women and couples—all of whom have access to free healthcare that the UK's National Health Service has to offer.

BEFORE I BEGIN, I want to reflect on my use of the word "baby" throughout this book, rather than "embryo" or "fetus." I realize that this could sit uncomfortably with the pro-choice arguments about abortion. Feminists have struggled with this tension: how to square their support for women's reproductive rights—including a right to choose abortion—with their desire to acknowledge and resolve women's reproductive suffering too, which includes their experience of losing a "baby" in miscarriage. Linda Layne, a US feminist anthropologist, reflects on this unease in her seminal book *Motherhood Lost*. She writes: "The fear, in the context of pregnancy loss, is that if one were to acknowledge that there was something of value lost, something worth grieving in a miscarriage, one would thereby automatically accede the inherent personhood of embryos and fetuses."

But I don't see it in quite the same way—and neither does Layne, who, like me, defines "personhood" (or "babyhood") as a notion that emerges from cultural, and individual, constructions. The women I speak with in therapy or elsewhere don't talk about the "inherent personhood" of what they have lost; neither do they claim that their own

particular relationship with their unborn is universal. I
know of women who experience the loss of established
pregnancies with little heartache or may find a miscarriage a
relief—and who don't use the word "baby" to describe what
they lost. And I know that feelings may change over time
too: a miscarriage can be a relief for a while but mourned at
a later date, just as the desired termination of an unwanted
pregnancy can later become a devastating loss.

But the word "baby" here also highlights how the English language shackles us when it comes to writing or
talking about miscarriage. Some English-speaking women
recruit words from other languages to capture their loss: the
indigenous Maori of New Zealand call a preborn child
"*pepi*" (referring to someone who has agency and can decide
whether to stay in or leave the womb), and Japanese Bud-
dhists have the word "*mizuko*," or water baby, who exists in
an in-between space between life and death, waiting to be
guided back into life at another time. But for this book, I use
"baby," as it's the one I most often hear from the bereaved.

AS I HOPE you will discover, every miscarriage is tethered to
its own meaning. I want the chapters that follow to help
equip you to think more deeply about what miscarriage
could involve, so that you in turn are able to talk about it
more easily. For those who already know what a miscarriage
can entail, I hope these stories both console and offer support for what remains a stubbornly marooned experience.
Although I acknowledge how far we have come, I also want
to show you how much further we can, and must, go.

The Brink *of* Being

One

A Child in Mind

THE UNCONCEIVED, BARELY CONCEIVED, UNUSUALLY CONCEIVED

> When you think you're pregnant, and you're
> not, what happens to the child that has already
> formed in your mind? You keep it filed in a
> drawer of your consciousness, like a short story
> that wouldn't work after the opening lines.
>
> —Hilary Mantel, *Giving Up the Ghost*

Miscarriage often involves the loss of a unique relationship with a baby—a relationship that may have begun long before the baby was conceived, especially for those who have yearned for a baby for years and may have struggled to get pregnant. But the notion of a relationship existing with our unborn—however developed in the womb he or she may be—took a pitifully long while to grab the attention of medical and psychological research and can still be a fragile one for many. And if this bond isn't fully understood, the grief flowing from its dissipation when a pregnancy ends has little chance of a healthy expression.

From the beginnings of my desire to get pregnant, nearly a year before I conceived my twins, I played out a number of stories in my head that also stirred my heart. Sometimes my baby was a girl, sometimes it was a boy, sometimes it had grown into a child. I would drift into reveries of how I would guide a teenage son to be a feminist or encourage a daughter to embrace physical adventures in a way that I never had. It didn't stop there—I even imagined becoming a doting grandmother to my grown child's children.

In early 2002, I took my first pregnancy test. I had, at last, a reason to suspect that my dreams had come true as, tantalizingly, my bleeding had failed to arrive. I knew exactly how the test worked, but I still read and reread the instructions in the packet, worried that if I interpreted them wrongly, I would sabotage any chance of becoming a mother. I prayed to a God I no longer believed in for a second pink line to emerge in the teeny white plastic window of the wand. My fantasy baby, wedged tentatively but tenaciously in my mind for the many months I had been hoping and hoping, was about to become real—or not. And when the second line did appear, the bond with my baby in my mind instantly changed dimension.

These heartfelt imaginings I both enjoyed and worried about are often beyond our control. If our thoughts have an emotional charge—such as "I desperately want a baby" or "Maybe this month I'll be pregnant"—they can easily become tenacious. Trying to stop thinking about something that concerns—or threatens—us rarely works: the ruminative power of our mind is too forceful. I have yet to encounter anyone who wants to be pregnant and can successfully switch off their hopes, dreams, and fears about it, even if they try.

This mental labor in itself contributes to the sparks of a relationship with our unborn: the more we think, plan, day-dream, or dream dream about our longed-for baby, the deeper the grooves in our mind become. In neuroscience, this concept has been summed up by the phrase "Neurons that fire together, wire together," coined by a Canadian be-havioral psychologist, Donald Hebb, who proposed that the more we repeat a thought, feeling, or behavior, the stronger the neural connections in our brain become. And as these neural connections strengthen, the more we are prone to these thoughts, feelings, and behaviors.

Imagine learning that you have a very good chance of winning the lottery over the next few months. I challenge anyone not to think about—or find themselves thinking about—what they would do with their winnings. A real possibility, or *probability*, of something life changing can worm itself deep into our minds and hearts. And when a pregnancy is confirmed, this probability—and corollary re-lationship with an unborn—that had prevailed in mind then literally prevails in body, and in the world too.

CLAIRE CAME TO SEE ME in the wake of her first miscarriage at nine weeks, and she left me in no doubt about the strength of her feelings for the baby she was still yearning for. Many other people she had turned to couldn't seem to under-stand that, for Claire, it didn't matter how tiny it was or that she was unable to describe what it looked like. Her

connection to her baby had begun months before its conception, and she described her thirty-five days of being pregnant as the most meaningful days of her adult life. While she
never used the word "love" to signal how she felt about her
child-to-be, it seemed a fitting word to me.

Claire had been with her partner Will for five years before they decided to have a child. They had talked about
their future family during these years, but it had remained
happily abstract until they began to try to conceive. She had
wanted to be a mother since her childhood, and had assumed
this role would be hers ever since she cared for her "cuddlies"
as a little girl and, later, when she changed her brother's
diapers and soothed him when he cried.

At first the couple luxuriated in their plans for parenthood while also enjoying each other, their friends, their hol-
idays, and their careers. Their future baby emerged from the
edges of their minds and became a fleshed-out being who
could be considered with confidence, ease, and increasing
detail: names and parenting styles were discussed. But as the
first year of trying to conceive rolled into the second, Claire
became less convinced that a pregnancy was going to happen. She described how an increasing lack of confidence in
becoming a mother seeped out into a general lack of confidence at work and even among her friends.

As her imagined baby crawled away from the easy reach
she had assumed for it, Claire would think about it more and
more, however hard she tried not to—the neurons were fir-
ing together and wiring together. She became increasingly
consumed with a desire to get pregnant, and the couple
turned to the seemingly endless advice about how to boost

their fertility. They gave up alcohol and late nights, bought expensive vitamin supplements, and took up yoga to combat the stress of unfulfilled desires. Sex became less spontaneous and carefree, and more of a necessity around the time of Claire's ovulation, whether either of them was in the mood or not. Claire stayed home more, in part because she was feeling more withdrawn, but also to protect herself from witnessing other pregnancies.

Each time Claire's period arrived, it brought increasing sadness and disappointment, as well as an excruciating mix of hope for the next month and despair that the hope might be destroyed again. Writing about his and his wife's struggle to conceive their son many years ago, the journalist Jon Ronson described his wife's experience of her period's repeated arrival as that of an "empty coffin." Those moving words returned to me when I heard Claire talk about her own months of trying to conceive: for her too, each menstrual bleed hurt like a small death.

Just as the couple was about to make an appointment with their doctor to investigate their fertility health, Claire's period was unusually late for the first time. Being pregnant had become so desperately desired, yet so unreliable a notion to believe in, that Claire needed extra proof that the baby she had nurtured in her mind was now actually in her body. It seemed too good to be true. She took four pregnancy tests before believing it herself, and then sharing the news with Will. Each stick revealed the word "pregnant," and she held on to them, not knowing then that they would become the only physical links to her baby that she would be left with.

The months of heartache evaporated in the couple's

all-consuming joy: Claire's long-cherished fantasy baby now *really* existed in terms that others could understand. While she assimilated her unprecedented news, her bond with her baby crystallized into one she could really take hold of, and she could now more confidently play out her maternal instincts through nurturing her own body with its new, precious cargo. She bought a pregnancy book, began to explore pregnancy websites, and signed up for email bulletins—she wanted to know everything that she could about her new state of being, and of the being she was inextricably bound up with too. However tiny and unformed as her baby was at this stage, this had no bearing on the strength of what she felt.

CLAIRE COULD RELY on a simple piece of technology to swiftly and unambiguously diagnose her pregnancy—although she was in such disbelief that her dreams had come true that she repeated the test. After detecting the presence of the hormone human chorionic gonadotropin (HCG) in her urine, released after an embryo implants to the wall of the womb about six days after fertilization, her pregnancy test literally told her—by displaying the word "pregnant"—that she was a mother-to-be.

Claire took for granted all that she knew about conception—the release of her egg each month and the related bodily symptoms this would bring. She knew that it would provide half of the genetic material for her baby and that its fertilization would lead to the development of a human baby—and, she happily assumed, a live birth. Up until relatively recently, though, educated and middle-class women like Claire would not have had definitive knowledge of any of this, or of their pregnancies, until many weeks after a hunch. And for centuries, women who miscarried may have been unsure as to whether they had lost a baby at all.

It may well be that our ancestors' relationships to a baby in mind were different from those of a modern woman. Although there are descriptions of pregnancy—and its losses—in historical medical works and other written records, we don't know very much about how women *felt* about these experiences—or how they related to their unborn. We have so few records of women's inner worlds at these vulnerable times. The historian Suzannah Lipscomb noted, "Most of the women who have ever lived left no trace of their existence on the record of history. In sixteenth-century Europe, it is likely that no more than 5 per cent of women—at most—were literate; ordinary women left no letters, diaries, or notebooks in which they expressed what they felt or thought. For us, their voices are silent."

It may be that there is far more material in historical archives than we yet know about, but so far, the event of miscarriage in the past is a largely unexplored one. With small patches of exception, it tends to be subsumed into historical, anthropological, or sociological studies about pregnancy and childbirth. Until we learn more about our foremothers' private experiences of their pregnancies and early endings, we have to make some educated guesses based on what we know that they could have known.

There are some fascinating ideas about conception and pregnancy in ancient Greek Hippocratic medical texts that were influential for centuries—at least until early modern times. Three particular works—*On Generation*, *Nature of the Child*, and *Diseases of Women*—tell us the most, including that a woman's body was deemed to be "wetter" and more "sponge-like" in texture than a man's "hard," "firm," and "more constant" one. This idea seems to have stuck around to this day.

Echoing the thinking of the Greek philosopher and scientist Aristotle, these writings stated that conception happened when a male seed imposed itself successfully into a shapeless mass of female blood. If a woman's blood did not overwhelm the seed of a man, and there was no fault with the male seed, then a human form could ultimately develop from this mass. Women were often blamed for conceptions going wrong, so it's interesting that a male seed could also be deemed to be at fault. Pregnancies were diagnosed at "quickening," when a woman felt fetal movements (probably around sixteen weeks), with a male fetus apparently moving before a female could.

Following this Hippocratic thinking, anything lost through the vagina before quickening was not only not a baby but also deemed not human. What women lost was often described as a "uterine mole" that related to reproduction, while the Greek physician Soranus in the second century AD had a different view in his manual for the Romans, *Gynecology*. He saw "moles" as nothing to do with reproduction at all, linking them to ulcers or inflammation of the womb.

We don't know how women in classical times experienced the loss of these ambiguous "moles." The received wisdom of the time told them they hadn't lost a baby who they may have harbored in their dreams. If women's mental worlds were the same then as they are now, it may be that some challenged the standard medical views, knowing their body and its rhythms better than anyone else. We don't know if they thought a lost "mole" was the early inklings of their human child, which they may well have gone on to mourn.

Centuries later, when print culture expanded in seventeenth-century Europe and midwifery texts began to circulate—such as Nicholas Culpeper's *Directory for Midwives* (1651) and Jane Sharp's *The Midwives Book* (1671)—the diagnosis of a pregnancy still remained bathed in ambiguity. Some vivid depictions of pregnancy and suspected pregnancy in early eighteenth-century German and French texts echo the classical view that a woman's unborn child came into existence once it became animated enough to be sensed. But even this wasn't a watertight determination, as these sensations could be confused with the movements of "moles," colic, or wind.

One academic has suggested that during these early modern times, "until the birth of a live infant, there was no certain way to determine whether what a woman harbored within her was a child or rather, as one often-reprinted volume put it, 'a foul mass of flesh that comes to no perfection.'" What the modern reader may now suspect were miscarriages were often described as "blood curds," "wrong growths," or even "fleshy morsels"—words that sound pejorative to contemporary ears but are sadly not so far away from phrases I've heard used in reference to a miscarriage in modern times.

We are unlikely to ever know if "fleshy morsels" might have been fondly dreamed-of babies to early modern women in the privacy of their own minds. Or whether such women followed other wisdom. But as pregnancy testing became more accurate—and more available—as the twentieth century progressed, they could become more confident about knowing about, and bonding with, their suspected child in mind.

Beginning in the late 1920s, laboratory tests were developed to detect a pregnancy: women's urine was injected into living animals (first mice and rabbits, then frogs and toads), whose resulting physiological changes from the HCG (or lack thereof) would indicate a pregnancy. But this cumbersome method wasn't available to all: doctors rejected "curiosity" cases of healthy married women, and testing became mainstream only when home pregnancy kits emerged on the market in the UK and US in the early 1970s. Although these now remarkably sensitive tests have largely removed any ambiguity around conception (false results do rarely occur), when it comes to a pregnancy then ending in miscarriage, ambiguity seems to linger around what the pregnancy created: we don't tend to know if a "baby" existed, as we don't tend to ask.

Imagery of life in the womb has also had a profound bearing on how women relate to their unborn. Many stunning depictions survive from the sixteenth century, such as Leonardo da Vinci's annotated *Studies of the Fetus in the Womb*, as well as awkward birth "presentations" (showing which part of the baby first enters the birth canal) that were published by the physicians Rösslin and Rüff and reproduced in midwifery manuals in premodern Europe. But these drawings would not have been mainstream, and images of less developed babies in the womb—those at risk of miscarrying—are far more of a modern phenomenon.

A new iconography began when the Swedish photographer Lennart Nilsson's photograph of an eighteen-week-old baby was published on the cover of *Life* magazine in 1965. The powerful cover image, and the accompanying photo story inside—"Drama of Life Before Birth"—plainly laid out the sophistication of human development from the moment of conception. It provoked heated debates about the beginnings of life and the status of the unborn, but also created new depictions for the mind's eye and expectant parents' hearts.

The bodies of babies growing in the womb have since been featured on other magazine covers, in advertising campaigns, and in art exhibitions. Invariably they fly solo: there is no sense of a womb cocooning these bodies, apart from an umbilical cord drifting off into the distance, like an astronaut attached to its mothership. This visual message of apparent autonomy may well serve to encourage our relationship with our unborn too: it suggests a being to be related *to*, rather than one that is an integral part of a woman's body.

CLAIRE WAS BORN INTO A world of this familiar imagery, and she saw it in her pregnancy book, on websites, and in the weekly email alerts she had excitedly signed up for. All of this would flesh out her unborn's unfolding persona, just as its body was literally fleshing out inside her womb. Two weeks after she took her pregnancy tests, she read about "Your Baby at Week 6" and the development of its "adorable face": "And are those little indentations on both sides of the head the sweet dimples you always hoped your baby would inherit . . . ? No, they're ear canals in the making."

Reading and rereading these tender, maternal words, which were accompanied by an image of a tiny human in the making, meant Claire began to feel a force of affection that she hadn't felt before. She began to wonder which features it would inherit from her and Will—although she told me that she never considered dimples. It was also around this time that another dimension of Claire's early pregnancy served to bind her with her baby: the visceral and relentless symptoms she endured.

Like many pregnant women, Claire began to suffer a daily rising tide of debilitating nausea and exhaustion. She felt so unwell that she could barely eat anything other than crackers and bread, and she would return each day from work only to fall asleep. Her sense of smell became acute, and her breasts painfully tender; even if her mind could briefly forget about the activity in her womb, her body would swiftly remind her. The author Rachel Cusk describes this visceral bind so well in her memoir about her first pregnancy and early motherhood: "In pregnancy, the life of the body and the life of the mind abandon the effort of distinctness and become fatally and historically intertwined."

Though the research is unclear on the matter, Claire had heard somewhere that her sickness was a sign of a healthy pregnancy, so as much as she detested her symptoms, she believed they were a price worth paying for becoming a mother. I can relate to this: my own still-memorable nausea put wind in my sails during my first pregnancy and gave me confidence to pad out my dreams. And like Claire, I took my suffering as a form of maternal duty that I felt privileged to have.

Even though Claire continued to gather as much information about her baby as she could, she had no way of knowing whether it was a boy or a girl at this stage. Her first routine scan (generally around twelve weeks in the UK) could offer a guess, but this would be more certain at her second scan, two months after that. But like some other women, she had a strong hunch and spoke of knowing that she was having a daughter from those early days. It was deeply moving to hear how nuanced her connection with her baby had become.

"I just knew it was a girl," she reflected. "While we were trying to conceive, I had a recurring dream about a child, and it was always a girl. Sometimes she was a toddler, sometimes a bit older. But they stopped after I found out I was pregnant—I like to think it was because she'd chosen to leave my dreams and come into the world. Will even had a name for her—Maggie—after his grandma who he adored. I would talk to Maggie every day, sometimes out loud."

Claire's pregnancy dreams and Will's choice of name from a family member reminded me of an Australian Aboriginal myth in which spirit-children are dotted around in caves, rocks, trees, and sand hills. They can take the form of animals, birds, or humans and can enter a mother's womb in a number of ways, such as appearing to a man in his dreams. After this nighttime appearance, the spirit-child can then enter his wife through her stomach, thumbnail, or foot. Sometimes, though, a spirit-child from an animal or bird enters a human mother, dooming the pregnancy to miscarriage. Claire's connection with her spirit-child was not just hers; Will would put his head on her belly at night and talk to Maggie, just as Claire did.

There were many ways in which Maggie embedded herself into the couple's present and future world, widening the contours of the small family's relationship as the days went on. Their dreams for Maggie's future went as far ahead as her schooling and her role as the eldest sibling. Plans for nearer times were more concrete: although Christmas was seven months away when Claire's pregnancy was confirmed, the couple had begun to think about how they would spend it, given Maggie's imminent birth. Claire's mother had moved to Spain years before, and they usually joined her there for festive celebrations in the warmth. But Claire assumed that she would be too pregnant to fly, so they spoke of different plans for a family celebration at their own home instead.

Claire's mother was equally excited by the idea, and offered to stay on after Christmas for a few weeks to help after the birth. "We were already thinking that we could ask for presents for the baby," Claire said. "I saw myself waddling around with a huge belly and enjoying the start of my maternity leave. It would be my first alcohol-free Christmas for years too." Although I didn't know, my guess is the memories of these Christmas dreams would have thrown a veil of sadness over that time, when it came around, for Claire, Will, and Claire's mother.

Just as Claire's mother felt protective of her daughter's new state, Claire felt her own protectiveness. Some of this was the product of her bond, of course, but her concerns also derived from cultural messages that it was her duty to protect her baby. She bought expensive pregnancy vitamins and avoided anything she perceived to be a risk to her pregnancy—regardless of what the research said. She turned down an arduous fund-raising swim and became nervous about her daily commute to work on a bicycle. "I was so careful about everything I did and everything I swallowed. I even worried about getting angry or upset. I didn't want the baby to feel my negative feelings, and I would apologize to her if I did get stressed."

In Korea, the traditional practice of Taegyo remains influential to this day. It rests on the idea that life begins at conception, and sets out recommended behaviors, thoughts, and even intentions that a mother should adopt to ensure the best foundations for her growing baby. As well as eating healthy food and avoiding orthodox medication (as opposed to traditional herbs), a pregnant woman is duty bound to educate herself further and, what must be the greatest challenge of all, to keep a peaceful state of mind—just what Claire strived for.

Our own Western culture also conveys powerful messages about responsible pregnancy, which Claire was clearly succumbing to and which bound her to a particular duty of care toward her unborn Maggie. Cusk writes about this too in her memoir, noting the iron rod ruling a pregnant woman: "I have been tagged, as if electronically, by pregnancy. My womanly movements are being closely monitored." Her caution about Maggie's safety meant she would place her arms protectively around her abdomen in crowds—she never forgot what was inside of her.

For the next couple of weeks of illness and preoccupation, Claire's bond with her growing baby continued to flourish. Her online update "Your Baby at Week 9" jauntily told her that her "medium green olive"–sized baby was developing tiny muscles to allow for spontaneous movements of its arms and legs, and also that "you won't feel your tiny dancer for at least another month or two."

But a couple days after reading about Maggie's limb movements, Claire noticed some small marks of blood in her pajamas one morning. She was not overly concerned, knowing from her voracious reading that spotting was not unusual in early pregnancy. But by the time she left work that day, she had become terrified: the bleeding was heavier, and she began to feel some mild cramps in her womb. She took herself to bed and left a message for her doctor.

Her detailed plans for Maggie's existence had become frighteningly precarious, but certainty about her fate came far sooner than Claire expected. Shortly after Will returned from work, her symptoms escalated. Her bleeding increased and the pain became unbearable. With Will's help, she struggled to the loo—the only obvious place for her copious blood to go. "I had no idea what more to expect, so I stayed sitting on the loo until nothing more came out of me," she told me. In a panic, she then flushed its contents away.

Claire hadn't felt her baby inside her during her precious weeks of pregnancy, nor could she be sure exactly when it was pushed out of her body into the water below her, because, at nine weeks, it was too small. Neither she nor Will had seen Maggie on an ultrasound screen—an experience that, research suggests, may have strengthened her bond even more. But there's no doubt that the size of her loss had no correlation with the tiny size of her baby—the dreams, plans, and hopes that had lived in her mind and heart amounted to far, far more.

At first Claire was in shock as her body and mind adjusted to a new way of being: she was no longer pregnant, yet she felt so very far away from her pre-pregnant state. She moved between a numbness and a crippling sadness for the enormity of what she, and Will, had suddenly been denied. Claire told me that she had received sympathy from friends and family, but it was largely short-lived, and her friends expected her to bounce back within days. "It was a bit like it was when I fell off my bike a few years ago—people realized it was horrid, but then quickly focused on the fact that I was okay." No one took the time to ask her—or Will—what Maggie meant to them; nor did anyone try to find out the size and shape of the hole in her life that her miscarriage had left. No one even asked if Claire's baby had a name.

Many people struggled with the extent of babyhood Maggie represented at such an early stage of gestation, echoing some of the historical negotiations around pregnancy diagnosis that we assume we have long left behind. One friend suggested to Claire that she must be relieved that "it happened early on, you know, before it developed into something." And just as I had keenly felt after my miscarriages, Claire also felt pressured to leave Maggie's memory behind—by getting pregnant again or by concentrating on other things. But the relationship she had forged would live on regardless, and therapy with me offered her a safe space for this reality to be fully grasped.

In my work with Claire, I took for granted what I know so well from my personal and professional experience: that the potential strength of a relationship with a baby who was only recently conceived can be formidable, and the source of a profound grief. Not everyone understands this, though— and it has taken a wretchedly long while for both our research community and our culture to begin to do so. There is an entrenched belief that a bond with a child can only really begin after a familiar-looking baby is born alive, and we still have a way to go before it fully dissipates.

UNTIL THE 1980S, there was a tragic lack of research interest into the psychological and emotional impact of the loss of a baby during pregnancy or during or after birth. Women had long been expected to endure all sorts of pain and suffering as an intrinsic part of their reproductive lot, and the loss of a baby at any gestation was a part of this. But miscarriages were also silenced and ignored, because it was assumed that a woman couldn't bond with her unborn baby in the way that she actually can, and does. And while it may have been conceded she might be more upset if a baby died later on in gestation, it was long thought that a woman shouldn't really grieve for a pregnancy that hadn't confidently established itself.

One of the first influential research papers on the subject of a woman's relationship with her unborn was published only a couple of years before I was born, in 1970. Its authors, Kennell, Slyter, and Klaus, wrote about the responses of mothers of babies who had died at birth, and suggested that their obvious grief provided evidence that a relationship could exist between a woman and her baby during pregnancy. Its summary paragraph states, with a subtle note of surprise, that of the twenty women interviewed after the death of their newborns, "every mother mourned even when her baby was nonviable and lived for only an hour."

Around the same time, two physician-psychoanalysts at London's Tavistock Clinic, Emanuel Lewis and Stanford Bourne, began publishing a number of articles in medical journals about their concern for the emotional health—and wish for better care—of women who lost their babies at birth. Although they explicitly cautioned that miscarriage shouldn't be "magnified into a catastrophe," believing that a woman's resilience after an early loss would be greater, their pioneering and compassionate work paved the way for new thinking about how women related to their unborn babies of all gestations.

As part of Bourne's research, he sent out a questionnaire to doctors who had attended both live and stillbirths, asking for simple "yes" or "no" answers to questions about their patients' responses, reactions, progress, and psychological history. What struck him most from the answers he received was the effect of stillbirths on his professional colleagues, along with "the disturbed doctor-patient relationship ensuing in these cases, characterised by a strong reluctance of doctors to know, notice or remember anything about the patient who has had a stillbirth."

Bourne deeply regretted the "professional deafness, blindness, and amnesia" of his colleagues, guessing that they were insufficiently prepared for these tragedies, which ultimately led them to be repelled by them. His observations remain relevant to miscarriage care and support today: we tend to avoid thinking deeply about it partly because we don't educate ourselves or prepare properly—and this includes some medical staff. In some medical settings, there are efforts to train health-care staff who treat pregnancies under threat, and charities offer their own trainings when hospitals can't (or won't) offer any.

While the tide slowly began to turn toward more appropriate thinking around the psychological experience of pregnancy in the eighties—including the notion that a woman could bond with a baby who was yet to be born—language that can be described as insensitive at best, tormenting at worst, was still being used in obstetric medicine. Pregnancy losses were sometimes written about as "fetal wastage," and a delivered dead baby of any gestation could be routinely described as "it." Even less humanity was given to babies with developmental problems in the womb: the word "monster" stings women I have spoken with to this day—an unpleasant topic I return to in another story.

But by the time Claire had her miscarriage, in the 2010s, the field of research into its potential emotional impact had, thankfully, broadened dramatically. This research was inspired by concerned medical staff and by the campaign work of influential pregnancy-loss charities, on both sides of the Atlantic (such as Sands, the Miscarriage Association, and Share). It was also prompted by calls from feminists to take women's reproductive experiences more seriously. Beginning in the 1980s, more and more studies exploring aspects of the experience of miscarriage were published, a trend that continues today.

We now have a valuable bank of contemporary psychological research that maps out and measures the possible consequences of miscarriage (the so-called psychological sequelae), including grief, anxiety, depression, and, more recently, the possible symptoms and diagnosis of post-traumatic stress disorder. Emerging anthropology, nursing, and psychotherapy literature signals an increased interest in understanding the lived experience of miscarriage in a number of different contexts too, although the research bank is far from full, and large gaps in its vaults still remain.

It's fair to say that clinicians are acknowledging and understanding the psychological aftermath of miscarriage more and more, which, in turn, can help them to adequately support the bereaved. But these inquiries don't—and can't—explicitly name a severed relationship with an unborn in the same way that the death of a child, or other loved one, may. Acknowledging the mental health suffering in the wake of miscarriage is vital, but it accompanies a reluctance to talk about lost motherhood or dead babies, as these are notions we can't define without considerations of cultural context, governing laws, and the range of individual responses.

Each relationship between a parent-to-be and his or her unborn is unique. Claire's relationship with Maggie would never replicate that of another one of my clients with her own unborn, nor would it be the same as the relationship Claire would have with her next baby in mind. And for some, this relationship may not even exist at all, even if they experience anxiety, depression, and trauma after a miscarriage nonetheless.

While I was thinking about the nuance and the potential psychological and emotional power of a child in mind, I wondered if it could also literally be detected by changes in a pregnant woman's brain. Many psychotherapists are excited by the developments of neuroscience, especially with its ongoing pursuit of demystifying the relationship between our intangible and often unfathomable minds to our tangible, jellylike brain. We are keen to learn as much we can about the physiological changes that can occur in our brains and bodily systems as a result of mental and emotional experiences, as this, in turn, can influence how we think about treating distress.

For example, we are discovering more and more about the influence of early parental care on our brain and hormonal mechanisms—and that these are partly measurable via MRI scans and blood screens. Knowing about these developments, I was curious to find out if a pregnant woman's mind could somehow map a relationship with her unborn onto her own brain. If so, this could demonstrate the impact of early pregnancy on a psyche in tangible terms—or at least add more material to the notion that pregnancy isn't just a "neck down" experience.

Until MRI scans for pregnant women are deemed safe enough for research purposes, we can't possibly know for sure what goes on in a pregnant brain—although I found a study that suggests we may have begun on this path. In early 2017, a team of researchers scanned the brains of twenty-five first-time mothers by MRI before and after pregnancy. The results showed pronounced changes in the structure of their brains—in particular, a significant reduction in gray-matter volume, which also happens in adolescence, suggesting a similar pruning away of weak synapses to make room for better ones. The data offers preliminary support for the idea that this pruning helps with the transition to motherhood, through encouraging necessary social skills.

But the few women in the trial who miscarried showed no such gray-matter changes, and the data suggests that the observed brain pruning happens late in pregnancy, and probably after birth too. Disappointingly for me, Claire's Maggie in her mind would have no observed neural correlates. But intrigued by all of this, I talked to one of the researchers. We wondered together about whether MRI technology would become sophisticated enough to both scan pregnant women safely (apparently, this is imminent) and also detect other brain changes early on in pregnancy that we can't yet see.

While psychological sequelae of miscarriage only *point toward* a relationship with an unborn, and brain changes in early pregnancy remain elusive, there is another field of psychological inquiry, attachment theory, that has attempted to measure the existence and quality of a relationship between a mother and her unborn. But this research largely informs the latter weeks of pregnancy, after twenty-four weeks—when miscarriages can't, technically, happen. This notion of prenatal attachment is an important one for the reasons I go on to describe, but it may also unwittingly serve to emphasize the strength of the bond with an unborn as it edges toward birth—at the expense of the bond with babies lost, far sooner and more frequently, to miscarriage.

Originally devised by John Bowlby in the late 1960s, attachment theory tells us that our early relationships with our caregivers have a profound effect on how we relate to others as we grow up, and into adulthood. If all goes well from birth, and we feel secure and loved and understood, this helps us successfully navigate our relationships—and our bereavements—as life unfolds. However, if we experience neglect or abuse early on, our probable resulting insecure attachments may set us up to struggle in relationships—and bereavements—that inevitably follow.

Prenatal attachment looks at the bond between a mother and her baby in the other direction, and departs from Bowlby's thinking in many other ways too. Its original impetus lay with the idea that if we can identify mothers at risk of not bonding with their babies during pregnancy, we may be able to help them develop nurturing feelings both before and after the baby's birth.

A handful of instruments have been devised to measure this bonding with our unborn, each named after its creator, including Cranley's Maternal-Fetal Attachment Scale, Muller's Prenatal Attachment Inventory, and Condon's Maternal Antenatal Attachment Scale. Cranley's instrument (devised in 1981) is probably the most commonly used and was originally based on six aspects of a pregnant mother's world: "differentiation of self from fetus," "interaction with the fetus," "attributing characteristics to the fetus," "giving of self," "role-taking," and "nesting" (although this last component was later dropped).

No hard conclusions from the studies using these scales have yet been drawn, apart from the fact that a relationship between a mother and her unborn does exist (later on, studies pursued this bond with the baby's father), and that this bond seems to strengthen over time as gestation progresses. We don't yet have enough evidence for prenatal attachment to our unborn in the first twelve weeks of pregnancy, when a miscarriage is most likely to happen, but my experience of talking to women like Claire tells me that their thoughts and behaviors could evidence most, if not all six, of Cranley's measurements.

More research needs to be done about the nature of our potentially powerful attachments to our unborn before and early on in pregnancy. This could be through an extension of prenatal attachment work, or through other research inquiries—brain scans are unlikely to help in the immediate future. But unless and until this happens, we can all do much of what I can do in my consulting room: be curious to discover the particular meaning of a miscarriage for the bereaved. I know that this will be a far more effective way of discovering the entirety of what has been lost than a sympathetic "I'm sorry" on its own.

A WILLINGNESS TO accept the powerful existence of a child held in mind may be even more necessary after more unusual experiences of losing an unborn—such as in the extremely rare cases of imagined pregnancies, the far less rare cases of molar and ectopic pregnancies, or IVF cycles that either fail or leave unused and loved embryos behind. In these cases, not only can the lack of a straightforward conception challenge the entrenched cultural idea of a baby, but the medical interventions they involve may also serve to overshadow the emotional experience of loss.

Although much of Claire's continued sadness and yearning was tangled up in her lost imaginings, she knew that she hadn't imagined her pregnancy: her shop-bought pregnancy test had proved it, after all. It would be unusual, given her context and culture, if not odd, for her to have believed in a pregnancy that hadn't actually happened to her—which is why, as a young child, I became fascinated by the case of one very famous non-pregnancy: that of Queen Mary I, wife of Philip II of Spain.

In 1554, at age thirty-eight, Queen Mary experienced what is now commonly known as a phantom pregnancy. She seemed to sincerely believe in—and yearn for—the arrival of a royal baby that never became real. According to her biographers, when Cardinal Pole greeted her with the same blessing Gabriel made to her namesake at the Annunciation, "Blessed art thou amongst women and blessed is the fruit of your womb," Mary's baby sprang to life inside her: she felt a quickening—movements—which, at that time, meant her baby gained a human soul.

Perhaps Mary became convinced of her pregnancy due to a combination of a deeply held religious conviction, the political pressure around her to produce an heir, as well as her own personal yearning to have a baby. Whatever the reasons, the effects were remarkable: her belly expanded and physicians attended to her sickness. As the months rolled on, preparations were made for the arrival of a prince or princess—his or her crib was beautifully carved, and Mary wrote letters of announcement in advance of the birth: she left the date blank and enough space after writing "*fil*" (son) to add the "*le*" (daughter) if she gave birth to a girl. She even prepared her will in case childbirth killed her—a common practice of the time.

Around her due date, news leaked out that a baby boy had been born, and celebrations filled the streets; bonfires were lit and joyful processions made. But no baby had been born. Mary's baby seems to have been real in her mind alone. Historians have debated the reasons behind this famous nonevent—perhaps it was an elaborate plan to keep her husband, Philip, by her side, or she had an ovarian tumor or cyst, or lacked menstrual bleeding as she approached an early menopause. Maybe she had lost a baby after all, but attempted to avoid her anguish by persisting in its denial.

Of course none of these possible reasons occurred to me as a young schoolgirl, nor was I taught about her experience through any sympathetic lens. The narrative was about a "madness" of believing in something so wildly out of touch with reality. As an adult knowing only too well about reproductive loss, I hate to think of the humiliation Mary must have felt at emerging from her confinement empty armed, and I also dread to think of the profound grief she may have endured.

Mary, who went on to have another imagined pregnancy two years later, isn't the only recorded instance of an early modern woman expecting a baby that never arrived. Clinicians today describe her case as one of pseudocyesis and often link her story with references to twelve different such cases in the Hippocratic writings of 300 BC or the case of "hysterical" Anna O written about by Freud, who believed she had conceived a child with her previous psychoanalyst, Josef Breuer. This phenomenon is scarcely recorded in the developed world today (nor is the allied experience of "delusion of pregnancy," where no physical symptoms exist), and we have yet to fully understand how it is a woman's mind can so powerfully affect her body's systems.

Unreal pregnancies now tend to reside in the realm of detached or even amused fascination, but also in fiction as a powerful vehicle for exploring the desire to have a child, along with the agony of a grief for him or her not appearing. In Edward Albee's play *Who's Afraid of Virginia Woolf?*, Honey's "hysterical pregnancy"—"she blew up, and then she went down"—is a foundation for her obvious vulnerability and melancholy. But her famously warring hosts for the evening, George and Martha, took their mutually imagined parenthood even further than Honey did: they created a son who lived in their joint mind for years after Martha's nonexistent pregnancy and her nonexistent delivery of him. The grief of lost parenthood that infuses this play is one of the reasons for its lasting literary influence, but it also conveys the oft misunderstood power of love for children who are yearned for yet exist only in hearts and minds.

Pseudocyesis is still reported today in developing countries where the technology to diagnose pregnancies is lacking, and there is also a tremendous cultural and familial pressure on a woman to bear a child. In my professional capacity, I have never heard of a case outside of instances of psychosis, although I know well how fraught the relationship between a desire for pregnancy and the interpretation of bodily symptoms can be while women are trying to conceive.

Rather than hearing stories of women believing in a pregnancy that hasn't happened, I tend to hear stories about women defending themselves against a belief in a pregnancy when they have been trying to conceive for so long. Women I speak with can readily discount a delayed period, swollen breasts, or other possible signs of pregnancy if previous months of disappointment have become the norm, along with a repeated monthly loss of a much wanted baby in mind. This is why Claire took four pregnancy tests to assure herself that her longed-for dream had come true.

While in a phantom pregnancy a baby definitively doesn't exist, a similar phantomness can sometimes haunt pregnancies that develop in such a way that they cannot create a baby, and will inevitably involve a miscarriage. In the case of a molar or an ectopic pregnancy, the fact that a child in mind is a biologically impossible one may test some sympathies and understanding, and can also be swallowed up by the necessary medical encounter that they involve. But a bond with a future child doesn't always have to be bound up with the existence of a biologically possible baby, or its viability.

A molar pregnancy begins with an abnormal fertilization of an egg that implants in the womb, and it is very rare, affecting only about one in six hundred pregnancies. Rather than an embryo growing as it should, a so-called hydatidiform mole (meaning a fluid-filled mass of cells) does instead—we're not sure why. This tiny growth can unfold in two ways: into a partial mole, when two sperm fertilize an egg instead of one, so there is too much genetic material for an embryo to develop; or else a complete mole, when an egg cell with no genetic material is fertilized.

In either case, cells that should become the placenta develop too quickly and colonize the space where an embryo would normally grow. A very small number of these pregnancies (about 14 percent of complete moles and 1 percent of partial moles) pose an even greater threat to a woman's health. When molar cells burrow excessively into the womb (and become invasive moles), they develop into choriocarcinoma (or trophoblastic disease), a form of cancer, for which, thankfully, there is an almost 100 percent treatment success rate.

Molar pregnancies are of particular medical concern because of this small but not insignificant risk of cancer. After a diagnosis—during a routine scan or after a miscarriage—a woman can have weeks or even months of follow-up to ensure that her abnormally raised hormone levels return to normal. She may even have to endure chemotherapy if cancer was detected. This often means that not only does the belief in her baby become more precarious after a molar pregnancy is diagnosed, but the repeated and invasive medical intervention can swamp a woman's story of loss and heartache.

I have met only a handful of women who miscarried in this unusual way. One memorably described to me how she assimilated the news that her pregnancy wasn't what she'd understood it to be: "I went from being pregnant to not pregnant to then being made to wonder whether I had lost a baby at all. The doctors were talking in technical terms and suggested that my baby was just some sort of growth. But to me, it *was* my baby, whatever the textbooks said. I just say I had a miscarriage now, because it's too complicated to explain what had really happened."

In her moving story on the Miscarriage Association website, a woman named Jessica alludes to a similar confusion about the status of a pregnancy that turned out to be ectopic (meaning "out of place"). Here, an egg fertilizes successfully, but then goes on to implant where it can't thrive, outside of the womb—usually in a fallopian tube, and far more rarely elsewhere inside the body (in 3 to 5 percent of cases). This is thought to affect one to two in one hundred pregnancies in the UK. In Jessica's case, her symptoms of pain and blood loss turned into a life-threatening emergency, as the growth of her embryo nearly ruptured her fallopian tube. If this had happened without treatment, she would have died in about five minutes. Women have lost their lives while trying to create another one.

She writes about her feelings of envy and grief while she sits in a restaurant, near a mother handling her screaming baby. She wishes to be doing the same and reflects, "I sort-of had a baby once. It was about two centimetres long." Had Jessica's baby taken hold a little farther along its destined tracks and in the lining of her womb, it may have thrived—and, perhaps, felt less "sort of." Like a molar pregnancy, the nonviability of an ectopic pregnancy and the medical intervention it involves can eclipse the grief for the baby that never was and never could be.

Whatever the realness of what women and couples

mourn by medical or cultural standards, this doesn't really matter when it comes to the realness of a relationship with their baby and the heartache of it not manifesting. And as I've explored, a woman need not even be diagnosed with a pregnancy at all for this to happen. In the case of IVF (or the similar procedure of ICSI), couples now have knowledge of their potential babies animating in a petri dish weeks before knowing if they will become yearned-for family members. Their bond with these nearly invisible potentials can be profound too.

In vitro fertilization is an increasingly used intervention for the one in six couples who struggle to conceive, and the best known. In July 2018, it was estimated that more than 8 million IVF babies have been born worldwide to date. Making babies in this way is now well established and certainly less taboo—a far cry from the arrival of "Our Miracle called Louise," as the first "test tube baby," Louise Brown, was greeted by one newspaper headline in 1978. Louise's parents had been trying to conceive for nine years; it doesn't take much to imagine their joy at her birth.

Couples turn to IVF after months, if not years, of trying to conceive the child in their minds. A typical procedure involves a woman taking drugs to stimulate her ovaries to create more eggs than her natural cycle would. The resulting eggs are then removed from her body so they can be fertilized with sperm in a laboratory. Any viable embryos that are created are either transferred into the woman's womb or frozen for later use; if they are deemed without potential to make life they are destroyed or left to perish.

An embryo—closely observed by lab technicians for its

successful cell division—can be proof enough of a much-wanted child coming down to earth from the world of dreams, just as the word "pregnant" appearing in her four home pregnancy tests was for Claire. But if an embryo doesn't go on to implant in a womb—an unfortunately oft-called IVF "failure"—its loss can result in utterly devastating grief, just like miscarriage.

The poet Julia Copus wrote about the stages involved in her IVF cycle in a sequence of exquisite poems titled "Ghost." It is to her that I owe the title of this book. In "Egg" she reflects on her embryo transfer, noting how the embryologist entering the treatment room, scrub cap on her head, looks similar to a bakery girl at Sainsbury's: "except instead of the iced buns she is carrying / the world's two smallest humans, deftly clinging / to the edge of her pipette, the brink of being."

Powerful feelings for our smallest humans are also closely examined in the moving and important play *The Quiet House*, in which Gareth Farr dramatizes one couple's journey through infertility and IVF. We witness Jess and Dylan's lives fall apart as they endure the agony of losing their imagined baby each month, while they simultaneously witness their neighbor struggle with, and complain about, the exhaustion of looking after her newborn baby. We bear witness to the excruciating steps their IVF procedure involves, as each one hangs in the balance of being a good or bad result.

We also learn how the couple's embryos are thought about as potential children. One scene opens with them awaiting a call from the clinic. By this stage of the play, we know that Dylan answers the calls—he takes as large a role as he can in a process that involves so many medical intrusions into Jess's body. This time, he finds out how the couple's embryos developed in the laboratory, a few days after fertilization, relaying the news to Jess that "five little lives" were created, while one of their embryos wasn't viable. Jess interprets this embryo as having "died," before willing the others to be "alive" the next day.

Dylan: They will be.

Jess: Jesus. I hate that they are in a lab somewhere. It feels wrong. I'm scared. I want to be with them. Is it weird if I go there?

Dylan: A bit.

Jess: Our children are in a Petri dish. That's mental. What if someone drops it?

Jess and Dylan aren't alone in using words such as "alive," "children," and "died" in reference to their embryos; nor is Jess "weird" for wanting to be with them. Other tender, protective, parental, and remarkable words about IVF embryos litter online threads among the fertility community: #embies, or their frozen siblings, #snowbabies and #frosties, are all cheered on and urged to take root in the womb and become babies who breathe the air that we breathe. Even the odd #cellfie, an image of life at a few cells old, makes its way online. It's clear here that neither "life" nor "death" in the human experience has to rest on a consciousness—nor an embodiment of any sort.

One colleague of mine had IVF nearly fifteen years ago.

Three embryos were created and she gave each one a name—they still trip off her tongue with great ease. Two were transferred back into her womb, while the other was left to perish as it was deemed not good enough quality. She didn't become pregnant—her two embryos didn't implant—but speaking with her makes it clear how deeply she felt toward her microscopic potential children. She still wonders if her abandoned, and named, embryo "was a little fighter" who would have made it after all.

Like my colleague, my client Sarah developed powerful feelings for her embryos. She sought my help to think about what she should do with the supernumerary ones that her final IVF cycle had created. She and her husband were in their mid-forties when we met, and their twin daughters were soon to start school. They were conceived after multiple fertility procedures, leaving two embryos that had been good enough quality to freeze. Sarah clearly felt protective over her snowbabies, although our conversations suggested more profound feelings too—amounting, in my view, to a maternal love. Her husband didn't feel the same: no attachment had stirred in him, so she faced her dilemma alone.

What we do with embryos that are not needed—disposition decisions—will vary according to the legal and clinical regimes where you live. At the time of writing, in the UK you have the option of keeping them frozen in liquid nitrogen for a total of ten years (although extension to fifty-five years is possible), donating them to another woman or couple, or donating them for approved research purposes. Freezing them cost money and nagged away at Sarah's conscience: "I often look at the girls and think about their genetic siblings. What would our family look like if their beginnings were in the freezer now and the frozen embryos were grown into other twins? When I get caught up in this, it makes it so difficult to let them go."

In order to make a decision, Sarah did what most of my clients do: plenty of online research and chatting to women in similar situations—those in the same predicament seemed to understand best. She stumbled across the little-publicized and little-known practice of compassionate transfer, which refers to the placing of embryos that won't be used for donation or IVF into a woman's vagina or womb. This placement is deliberately done when there is no risk of a pregnancy occurring—either because of the timing of a menstrual cycle or because a woman has had her menopause.

This option of disposition appealed to Sarah, as allowing her twins' potential siblings to perish alone didn't sit comfortably with her maternal instincts, but such compassionate transfer was unavailable at her fertility clinic. RESOLVE: The National Infertility Association, in the US, lists it as one of the available options for IVF patients with unused frozen embryos, although not every clinic allows for it. Sarah conveyed her bond with her snowbabies with conviction: "I would like them to die where they could have died—not alone, but with me. It feels like a fair way of honoring them for offering us potential." It could even be said that Sarah was electing to have a sort of miscarriage.

Sarah's predicament would not have arisen without the rapidly evolving wonders of reproductive technologies, but it is also testament to the strength of a connection we can make with a child who may or may not even have been a

technical—or biological—possibility. In order to understand the anguish of miscarriage as best we can, we have to
take on board how the experience inextricably relates to this
nuanced, individual, and powerful tie that resides in the vast
privacy of a mind, not just a pregnant body.

Two

Derailed

EARLY MISCARRIAGE

I watched a rosebud very long . . .
Then, when I thought it should be strong,
It opened at the matin hour
And fell at even-song.

—Christina Rossetti, "Symbols"

My first pregnancy was fraught from the start, with repeated bouts of heavy bleeding—an obvious and terrifying symptom of a pregnancy undoing itself. It was no wonder that I feared having a miscarriage in those early weeks. We think the majority of miscarriages happen in the first trimester—before twelve weeks—and given that around one in four pregnancies end in miscarriage, I had good reason to fear the worst. But many women aren't like me. They don't expect it to happen and are not prepared for what it may involve: neither the potential physical—and possible medical—endurance nor the roller coaster of competing and complex feelings that the grief for a lost pregnancy can involve. The sadness, guilt, self-blame, sense of failure and worthlessness, anger, and uncomfortable envy can surprise or even shock the bereaved, who bear all this with no sure sense of how or how long to grieve, nor confidence to talk about an experience that has been relentlessly silenced.

"Early miscarriage" describes a broad range of experience: from the time when a pregnancy is confirmed until around three months later, when the implanted embryo has long become a fetus (this transition in status happens around eight weeks after conception). Research papers refer only to miscarriages in pregnancies that have been diagnosed medically (by ultrasound and/or blood test)—rather than suffered unreported—so it may even be that our estimates of incidence are slightly low. One hypothesis is that up to two-thirds of conceptions won't end up in a live birth, pointing to an undetectable phenomenon of a conception going awry before it implants in a womb, or soon after implantation, but before a menstrual bleed. For now the loss of these enigmatic inklings of life are untraceable, but perhaps they will be in years to come—just as our once-unfathomable pregnancies are so easily known to us now. I know that many would be mourned if detected.

An early miscarriage will always involve the loss of blood, and as the weeks progress, this is often far more blood—and far more pain—than a regular monthly period brings. More alarmingly for a woman, she may lose unrecognizable blood clots and placental tissues from her vagina, and also always, ultimately, her tiny baby too—whether naturally through her womb's processes, with a nudge from prescribed medication, or with surgical intervention. Sometimes, surgery needs to be repeated once or multiple times if it initially fails to remove all trace of the pregnancy. We tend to shy away in fear—and disgust—from knowing about these potentially traumatic and visceral aspects of loss, just as we shy away from knowing that an early miscarriage can cause a shattering type of grief.

LUCY, like many clients I have worked with, hadn't considered that a miscarriage could happen to her. She already had a two-year-old son, Freddie, and had happily sailed through each of the three potentially choppy seas of having a baby the first time: a quick conception, a full-term pregnancy, and a straightforward birth. So when she miscarried in the ninth week of her second pregnancy, she was shocked but also overwhelmed by her grief and all the sadness, anger, guilt, and envy that rolled around inside it. These feelings collided with each other at times, especially as she was desperately hoping to be pregnant again, while grieving the baby she had lost—and treasuring the living child that she had. When we first met, a couple of months after her miscarriage, she burst into tears before saying anything at all.

Although Lucy had undeniably suffered an enormous dose of bad luck, she was keen to tell me first about the good luck she recognized and enjoyed: like many other women after miscarriage, she wasn't sure if she could allow herself all of her distress. This was made more understandable given that many of the condolences she received from friends and family were framed by her good fortune: like "at least you have Freddie" or "thank goodness it happened early on" or "you have a wonderful marriage." She feared sounding ungrateful for what she did have, yet this also made it difficult for her to talk about what she had been deprived of.

Lucy had worked hard to nurture her unborn babies during both of her pregnancies, and I got to know her perfectionist streak well. We could trace this back to events in her childhood, but I could also see that she was succumbing to an overwhelming pressure about how to mother best, a burden that began even before her babies were conceived. Lucy's choices before and during both of her pregnancies were carefully considered: which folic acid to buy, which food or drink to consume, and even which hair dyes to use. She long planned for the natural birth she ended up having with Freddie, without pain relief or medical intervention, and persisted with breastfeeding despite his struggle to latch on, and the exhaustion she suffered because of it. This success/ fail binary lurking in conversations around mothering profoundly reiterated in Lucy's experience of loss.

Lucy's efforts to maximize her fertility were focused on a clear goal of creating her second child—she didn't think much about the possibility that it could die in the womb. I remember this blissful ignorance too: when I first tried to conceive, my repertoire of stories about pregnancy and birth barely included those of pregnancy loss. As a child, my mother told me about only one of her three miscarriages. She swiftly, quietly mentioned her loss as she parked a car outside the house of a friend we were visiting for lunch. But it remained a mystical, otherworldly event in my six-year-old mind and wasn't discussed again—nor the other two—until I lost my own babies. So pregnancy remained something magical—it produced babies—and then, at my senior school, it became an event to avoid at all costs.

My sex education as a teenager at school involved a cursory discussion on the necessity and use of contraception, accompanied by our biology textbook's cartoonlike images of a baby's development in the womb: a phenomenon that would occur if we didn't use protection. We were never told that conception could be difficult or impossible for one in six couples, or that pregnancy probably had a 25 percent chance of ending before twelve weeks, or that the risk of miscarriage creeps up significantly during the years we were supposed to be forging our careers. Campaigners in the UK are working hard to influence a new contemporary school curriculum that tackles these issues head-on: we need a new generation that is both better prepared for a dream to shatter and also more easily able to think and talk about reproductive loss.

When I did get pregnant for the first time, my borrowed, popular pregnancy bible didn't educate me well either. It briefly dealt with miscarriage toward the end of its walk through the three trimesters and birth, whereas I had repeatedly thumbed the early pages. Of course I didn't want to linger on the possibility that my growing babies could die inside me, but tackling miscarriage—and its aftermath—head-on in pregnancy literature and education may also be one small way to creating new, and easier, conversations. No one I knew then was having these conversations; nor do I hear many more now.

LUCY TOLD ME the story of her lost baby's life from its very beginnings in her mind. She and her partner, Cass, decided to try for another baby a year after Freddie was born: "We wanted two children close in age, and I was excited to do it all again with more confidence." She didn't expect to conceive as quickly as the first time, being thirty-five by then, but she was pregnant after the third month of trying. "We were both so excited! I was amazed that I'd conceived so easily again, and this set me up to assume the pregnancy was going to be like it was with Freddie—I'd be sick and tired for a while, and then I would feel great and really enjoy getting big." Sure enough, a couple of weeks after her pregnancy test, she began to suffer the same symptoms as before: exhaustion and nausea, with strange cravings, alongside nurturing her excited future plans.

Lucy and Cass happily gazed forward. They plotted out life with two young children—they needed to think about new child-care arrangements and to save up for a bigger car. Lucy bided her time through the illness, believing it would lift around her twelve-week scan, as it had with Freddie. "I limped through every day at work feeling dreadful—no one knew I was pregnant as I didn't want my boss to know I'd be taking another maternity leave quite yet. It didn't occur to me that something could go wrong; it just felt like it had before." But in the ninth week of her pregnancy, with no warning, Lucy woke up one morning with a clear sense that something had gone wrong.

"I woke up really early, feeling strange. I no longer felt

sick, and I felt a heaviness in my womb—I had never felt anything like it. I had been to hospital a week before for my booking-in appointment with a midwife, so I called the prenatal department as soon as it opened. Cass thought I was overreacting as I didn't have any symptoms, other than a sense of worry and mild dread." A midwife advised Lucy to call the early pregnancy unit if she experienced bleeding or pain, but otherwise to "sit tight and not worry, and that probably all was well."

Lucy wasn't soothed by these words—her hunch that something was awry was strong—but the views of the medical profession can have tremendous power in pregnant women's minds, especially in times of anxiety. Prenatal care is available to all pregnant women in the UK, and it offers extra checks, screenings, and resources in between regular appointments if need be. This is a wonderful privilege compared to many countries, yet I agree with the many women who think that the pregnancy—and indeed birth—experience has become overly medicalized and that their voice can be easily drowned out by protocols and procedures—and lack of time and staff.

But there is an ambivalence, and perhaps a paradox too: while we can resent overmedicalization and our compromised status as a patient rather than an individual, we also rely heavily on science and medicine to provide answers and offer solutions, and can rail against it when it fails to do either. And when it comes to miscarriage, we have every reason to rail: it is only relatively recently that research has prioritized tackling its causes and prevention, and many answers and solutions are still a very long way off. It's also only relatively recently that a woman's experience of miscarriage has come to be seen as a psychological as well as physical experience too.

Lucy had worked hard to rely on her intuition during Freddie's pregnancy and birth and this had rubbed up against medical opinion at times. She had campaigned not to be induced when Freddie's due date came and went, strongly believing he was safe despite the standard rules saying otherwise. She hadn't attended every antenatal appointment offered to her, preferring to rely on her body's knowledge. Hearing the midwife say "sit tight and don't worry" echoed these tensions between her own discernment and that of the medical voice that is heard in pregnancy and birth, and she was left frustrated by not being trusted more.

This sometimes fraught negotiation between a woman's wisdom of her pregnant body and that of a medical expert extends far back in time. The diagnosis of a "true" vs. "false" pregnancy was a vexed question for centuries, especially during the instances of women "pleading the belly" in defense of a crime in early modern European times. If a woman was deemed truly pregnant—as opposed to harboring a "false" molar pregnancy—she would avoid a death sentence, but it seems that in certain contexts the power could shift between herself and a medical expert. A woman's hunch that she was pregnant sometimes held sway in court, but not always—and women today like Lucy can still experience a similar variation in others' trust about what is going on in her womb. Sometimes women are listened to, but sometimes, regrettably, not.

After her conversation with the midwife, Lucy dropped

Freddie at day care and went to work, distracted by her fear of things getting worse. "The midwife's words ran around my head all day. I tried so hard not to think about my body, but of course I couldn't." Later that evening, as she was putting Freddie to bed, things did get worse: Lucy noticed a bloodstain on her trousers. "I then knew that something was wrong after all, but I also didn't want to believe it. I just didn't know whether to hope all was okay or not. Cass called my sister to come over and look after Freddie, and as the early pregnancy unit was shut, we had nowhere else to go but to accident and emergency."

It was a shame that Lucy's bleeding hadn't happened a few hours earlier, when she had a chance of being attended to by staff trained in threats to early pregnancy and their possible hazardous progression. Early pregnancy units began to proliferate in the UK in the 1990s, and tend to be a reliably compassionate place for worried parents-to-be. By contrast, accident and emergency is a medical setting unlikely to offer the most appropriate care for a threatened miscarriage, unless a woman's health is in serious jeopardy, such as with some ectopic pregnancies that may prove potentially fatal, or where there is seriously heavy blood loss. Emergency care is, by definition, geared toward rapid treatment of emergencies or lifesaving care to the ill or injured—not for a woman who was clinically safe like Lucy but terrified that her much-loved baby's life was under threat.

Luckily Lucy and Cass arrived on a Monday night—one of the quieter nights in a central urban A&E. Lucy was seen quite quickly by a triage nurse, but then had to wait for an attending doctor. He assessed her before calling for a

specialist, a gynecological doctor. The wait for a diagnosis—
and the need to repeat their story—while Lucy bled was
excruciating. "We were there for three hours before I was
properly examined. We were both sat on a bed in a tiny
cubicle with the curtains around us, holding hands while
unseen people screamed out in pain. It didn't feel right being
there. Cass looked for a spare chair, but there wasn't one. I
wasn't bleeding heavily then, but I was terrified it would get
worse and we didn't think to bring other clothes. We were
desperate to know what was going on. Eventually, a doctor
arrived. She was nice but brisk, and it seemed like she had
seen women like me a million times before."

After examining Lucy's softening cervix, the doctor
confirmed that her pregnancy was ending and said that it
was best that she go home to let "nature take its course."
There was no separate room for this devastating news to
be delivered in; nor did the hospital transfer Lucy to a
more appropriate ward, away from the trauma of the emergency department. The shocking diagnosis competed to be
heard among the sounds of machines going on and off and
strangers' voices—a memory that Lucy will always hold as
"surreal."

This so-called expectant management of early
miscarriage—allowing nature to take its course—is often
advised as a first course of action, especially in the initial
nine weeks of pregnancy. There was nothing anyone could
do to derail the inevitable, and after Lucy dressed herself
in her bloodied clothes, the doctor hurriedly described
what she was going to do next: make an appointment for a
follow-up scan and find Lucy a leaflet of advice. Lucy has a

fuzzy memory of this horrific episode, although she keenly remembers the doctor's emphasis on protocol and how she failed to say "I'm sorry."

"I was sobbing in Cass's arms, so I couldn't really take in anything she was saying to me. I wanted to know why, and I wanted to know what to expect. But she couldn't say how long it would take or how painful it could be. She seemed mostly concerned that I had to 'pass all the pregnancy tissue'—but I wasn't even sure what this meant. She didn't seem to register that our precious baby was dying or dead, and that we didn't even know which." Lucy and Cass were discharged with Tylenol and a scan appointment letter but no leaflet, as the doctor couldn't find one. Cass called a taxi and Lucy braced herself for what was to come.

Around 137,000 women in England each year experience pain and bleeding in early pregnancy and turn up for medical care in hospitals, and early pregnancy loss accounts for around 50,000 inpatient admissions in the UK each year. Comparable statistics in other countries are difficult to track down, partly because of the international variation in what constitutes early pregnancy, as well as the different ways in which patient records are taken and recorded. This lack of clear data hinders accurate comparisons being made for important research into miscarriage, and arouses frustration in the clinical community. But regardless of these ambiguous numbers, it is safe to say that emergency departments around the world treat pregnancies under apparent threat all too frequently.

Emergency departments are guided by treatment protocols that are primarily focused on acute care, large disasters, and accidents. They also offer "safety net" care for patients who aren't registered with a doctor or need help out of hours: they are invariably staffed by overstretched professionals. Unfortunately, like it did for Lucy, this means that a threatened, "straightforward" miscarriage can easily become treated as a routine medical event with no or little acknowledgment of the potentially desolating experience it can be. But for Lucy, her miscarriage *was* a life-and-death situation: it was the death of her baby, her child-to-be and sibling to Freddie.

Like the doctor who examined Lucy, staff in emergency departments who are faced with a threatened miscarriage are generally primed to rule out any immediate danger to a woman's physical health, and then decide on the best way to manage it if the loss of the pregnancy is inevitable. They aren't routinely trained to think much beyond this assessment—to consider, as protocol, the possible and potentially broad emotional impact of what a miscarriage can involve. Studies have shown that health-care professionals in emergency departments—like many people beyond hospital walls—can perceive the emotional needs of a miscarrying woman to be of far less importance than a woman after a stillbirth or neonatal loss. But just because these later losses involve differing treatment protocols—and would never involve a woman being sent home—this doesn't necessarily mean they exist in a different emotional realm.

A general practitioner talked to me about her training in gynecology fifteen years ago before she had her own two miscarriages: "When I worked in a busy London A&E, I could see up to eight or nine women presenting with a threatened miscarriage in one shift. If only I knew then what I know now about what it feels like to think, or know, that you are losing your baby. I would have considered those women differently." Thankfully, campaign work on both sides of the Atlantic since then has targeted a crucial need for better education around miscarriage care in emergency departments, with the National Perinatal Association in the USA, for example, urging patients like Lucy to be considered as experiencing a potential "emotional emergency"—with appropriate compassion, concern, and privacy—rather than a female body suffering a pregnancy complication. But this training has yet to become mainstream; nor are there resources for private rooms—and women like Lucy can often feel marginalized, ignored, or even forgotten.

Not only had Lucy been denied a compassionate response to the inevitable loss of her baby; she also lacked information about what to expect during and after her miscarriage—or even when it might happen. Being told to allow "nature to take its course" isn't good enough—she didn't know what this meant in literal terms or what was usual versus what she should be concerned by. She didn't know what her tiny baby would look like, whether she should or could retrieve it, how she could preserve it for a funeral rite, and what that could even involve. Nor did she know about the possible, excruciating level of pain to expect. The leaflet the doctor promised her failed to transpire—but even if it had, given the ones I have seen, it was unlikely to tell the whole visceral truth.

We all tend to flinch away from discussing the details of reproductive bodily functions, but I am often surprised by the tentative and euphemistic language that can be used by some medical staff too. The women I talk to prefer to know what a miscarriage will mean for them, without obscured or spared detail: you only have to read online miscarriage forum threads to see how much women rely on each other to plug the gaps in their knowledge about what happens to their bodies while and after pregnancies end too soon. Posts are often vivid in their depiction of the process (albeit premised with apologies for TMI) and questions about blood, clots, and pain abound, as do questions about future menstrual bleeds and when it is safe to be having sex again.

Lucy didn't go online to find the answers to her many unanswered questions, but over the course of the following day, her symptoms worsened, and her fear of what was coming next climbed. "I couldn't do anything but wait, in pain. It was hell on earth. And I had no idea how much it would hurt—I assumed that if I was given Tylenol it wouldn't be that bad, but it was horrific. I couldn't get comfortable, and I kept pacing around the bedroom and curling up on the bed when the pain hit hard. I remember thinking about my labor with Freddie, so I must have been comparing the two experiences. And then I suddenly felt something give way and a pressure bearing down on my cervix."

When she felt that her tiny baby's delivery was imminent, Lucy took herself to the bathroom, the only place she could think of. Cass, by her side throughout, followed her. Her sole preparation for the end of this second pregnancy was Freddie's birth, which she had both expected and planned in fine detail: she knew who would be there, where it would take place, what music she would listen to, and even what visualizations she wanted to practice to ride out the pain. Nothing could have prepared her for what was about to happen during her miscarriage though. "I sat on the loo, crying out in agony with Cass by my side. I then felt everything come out of me at once. I knew the moment when Freddie was born of course, but that day I couldn't tell what had been a part of me and what hadn't been a part of me. I don't even know if I can use the word 'birth.'" Nor, over time, would Lucy know whether to use the words "baby" or "mother" or "sibling" either.

Women often experience early miscarriages at home, in their bathroom, with no medical intervention—we'll never know how many, as no country keeps a register for such unhappy events. In fact, there is no official record for any baby lost under twenty-four weeks in the UK (which also makes sharper statistics difficult). Registration of a pre-twenty-four-week loss is an emotive and live issue in the UK, and my story about Emma and Jen in the next chapter explores this in some greater depth. But as I write, clinical guidance in the UK encourages "management" of early miscarriages at home, in an effort to reduce medical intervention where possible (unless there are clinical reasons otherwise or a previous trauma related to pregnancy).

Miscarriages can happen very quickly, as it did for Lucy, or they can drag out over days or even weeks. We don't tend to share hidden delivery stories such as these, but I make a point of being curious about these important moments, and I'm not sure that Lucy would have volunteered more detail had I not been so. "I knew when it was all over, but I wanted to be sure that the baby had come out. I put my hand in the loo and scooped up a small handful of bloody flesh. Cass didn't want to look, but I held it in my palm and studied it closely—there was a tiny sac with a baby in it, just a couple of centimeters long. I could see tiny legs, tiny arms, and an umbilical cord from its tummy. I kept asking Cass what the doctor meant by 'pregnancy tissue,' as what I held in my hand wasn't that."

Lucy would later berate herself for doing next what so many women do: "I panicked and dropped it back in the loo and flushed it away." But few women know what to do with the tiny bodies of babies that we lose to an early miscarriage, and Lucy hadn't been told that she might want to retrieve her baby for a funeral rite, and if so, how she could keep it safe. Furthermore, she didn't know that if she wanted to officially bury or cremate her baby, she would need a letter from a medical practitioner to confirm its miscarried status for a cemetery or crematorium. Lucy didn't know that she was free to bury her baby in her garden or elsewhere if she preferred. But even if she had known all of this, I doubt she would have found an easy place in her social world to discuss it with ease: burial rites tend to refer to the death of an established human life.

After Freddie was born, Cass cut his umbilical cord and a midwife passed him to Lucy for her to put him to her naked breast. She marveled at his familiarity and perfectly formed features. She counted his fingers and toes. Cass did too. But the baby Lucy held in the palm of her hand after her miscarriage looked very different from Freddie—a family resemblance couldn't yet be seen. I doubt Lucy shares her first memory of seeing her second baby with friends and family in the same way she does about Freddie, nor did she or Cass take a photo to capture these moments. We aren't used to seeing embryonic bodies, and Lucy was still troubled when she remembered how this intimate moment involved such a mixture of unbridled love, yet an unease too.

IT MAY BE that our disquiet with early developing bodies isn't modern. The seventeenth-century English author Lady Mary Carey left us with a number of beautiful writings that were inspired by her fear that she would die in childbirth. The longest of her prose poems, and the final one she wrote, in 1657, reflects on the miscarriage of her eighth baby, suffered eleven days earlier. It is very rare to find historical testimony about a woman's intimate feelings after such a loss, and the poem suggests she had no doubt that hers had been a human conception as opposed to a false pregnancy, as early pregnancies could then be suspected of being. After all, she was experienced in pregnancy. But like Lucy, her response to the disturbing sight of her tiny unformed baby was not straightforward, writing: "What Birth is this? a poore despised Creature? / A little Embryo? void of Life, & Feature."

In contrast to Lucy and Lady Mary Carey's hesitancy, a young woman, Nico, has posted nearly eight minutes of footage of her handling her eight-and-a-half-week-old baby on YouTube. She introduces it with the written comment: "This video is very TMI but I thought I'd share this Incase anyone would like to see where there baby is in growth." It was probably a week younger than Lucy's baby, and Nico handles its tiny body with remarkable confidence, not least because she tells us it came out of her own body twenty minutes before she began filming. She talks to the camera about her belief in it being a boy (she couldn't have known visually) before warning us, "Now I will show you the baby."

Carefully and tenderly, Nico points out the details of a complete gestational sac containing her "little guy" with its nascent limbs, obvious fingers, almost-toes, threadlike umbilical cord, early intestines, and eyes. Her warmth and directness make the footage moving viewing, and her "TMI" is clearly manageable for the more than half a million visitors who have so far watched at the time of my writing. Nico's affectionate, perhaps maternal, feelings seep through her speech, and I admire her candor in sharing an experience that sits far more comfortably out of cultural—and YouTube—sight.

Perhaps Nico's desire to educate her viewers gave her some solace in the wake of her loss: she could contrive some sort of purpose. Many women are keen to participate in contemporary miscarriage research trials for similar reasons, and we mustn't forget their crucial role in pushing the growth of much-needed knowledge ahead. It may also be that without women and their families willing to give their miscarried babies away in our past, we may not have advanced the field of embryology. One thought-provoking paper explores the invaluable contribution that some nineteenth-century middle-class American women made to this area of crucial research. While French and German embryologists were breaking new ground in European hospitals and laboratories, some researcher-physicians in America created a new site of scientific research—at the bedside of miscarrying women.

Letters and journals of this time record how women, confined to bed as their pregnancy ended, would hand over their miscarried babies to waiting physicians, who would pursue their research on their "specimens" elsewhere. It seems that these women could be relieved or even overjoyed at the whole event. Unlike Nico or Lucy, they had little in the way of reliable and safe contraception and may have birthed many children already. Framing their miscarriage as an experience that aided the new science of embryology may have been emotionally helpful to these women too— perhaps to make more sense out of the positivity they felt, when they were expected to be sad. But Lucy lives in a different time and a different place. She was the opposite of relieved, and unable to soothe herself in any way with an idea that her miscarriage could help further research.

LUCY'S GRIEF WAS ACUTE FOR weeks after the event she had described to me. She spoke of good days when she felt sad but able to carry on, with a hope of a return to her previous happiness. But there were also terrible days, when her yearning for her baby overwhelmed her: such as the day her twelve-week scan was due, and she'd imagined revealing her baby to her world, and a few days later, when she received a letter from the hospital noting that she hadn't turned up for her scan. This administrative blunder was a black-and-white reminder of a forgetting she frequently encountered and that angered her greatly. "I did get sympathy and kindness from the friends that we told, but it was all quickly forgotten. Ten days after, I took Freddie to a party, and no one mentioned a thing."

I still remember the DNA (did not attend) letters for various appointments that I received after my miscarriages, as well as the rage these mistakes provoked in me. Informing all hospital staff of a miscarriage, so that such appointment letters are canceled, has been another area of campaign work, and it seems that hospital staff are becoming more reliable at letting their colleagues know of pregnancies on their books that have ended. But errors still do happen, and, as Lucy experienced, they can be excruciating.

Despite feeling vulnerable, Lucy felt ready to try and get pregnant again—she still wanted to have another baby. She didn't want a baby to *replace* the one she had lost: she wanted another, different, baby who would live. And while Freddie was of great comfort to her, he wasn't a replacement for the baby she had lost either. Cass wanted to wait, as he could see how devastated she was, but Lucy was convinced that she was ready. But this also meant she felt guilty about seeming to leave the memory of her lost baby behind—along with feeling guilty for flushing it away as waste and for being distracted from Freddie.

Guilt, along with its close cousin self-blame, persists in the wake of most miscarriages—especially when it comes to trying to understand why it happened in the first place. Lucy believed she had somehow *caused* her miscarriage. But no one would know for sure why it had happened, not least because her baby's body hadn't been investigated in a postmortem. Even if Lucy had kept her baby's body and taken it to the hospital, it is extremely unlikely it would have been examined. Most miscarriages aren't investigated, and more than half of those that are (after "recurrent"—or three consecutive—miscarriages and a referral to a specialist clinic) will not be given a concrete cause. Sporadic miscarriage—the one-off type—is assumed to have most likely been caused by a physiological phenomenon as an embryo develops, meaning that some serious chromosomal problems or other structural malformations prevent it from thriving.

Random chromosomal errors just happen: some view human reproduction as inefficient; others that this kind of abnormality is a mechanism that allows us humans to space our pregnancies. A lapse between pregnancies can, the thinking goes, help parents offer "good enough" nurture to their infants, preventing the parents from being too wrung out with exhaustion, and for a woman to recover well after birth. There's also an idea that a baby born with development problems would suffer in life too, and many condolences for miscarriage draw on this idea of "nature's way." This potential higher wisdom didn't cancel out Lucy's grief though—nor could she ever be sure that her baby had been chromosomally abnormal.

Cognitive processing theories of psychology tell us how important meaning-making is while we attempt to adjust to stressful experiences. After any bereavement, we feel the need to ask "Why?" In the context of miscarriage, I nearly always hear women turn to themselves in the face of not knowing why—and they can be fantastically creative when they do. Explanations when they *are* given can be so helpful to hold on to, and while research laboratories are busy recruiting women and investigating the causes of miscarriage, we are still years away from offering them routinely.

Like so many women, Lucy found it far easier to attribute her loss to her own doing than anything else, and then punished herself with a battery of "shoulds": "I shouldn't have worked so hard. I was up and down a ladder the week before it happened, painting an enormous theater set. I should have worn a mask to protect me from the paint fumes. I should have ignored the midwife and gone to the hospital earlier." Lucy's personality meant that she easily turned against herself, but her logic is familiar to me nonetheless.

In Lady Mary Carey's case, her beautiful meditation on her loss reveals a similar self-punishing logic. She wrote—not intending it for publication—at a time of Protestantism that committed her to the all-seeing and guiding nature of God, and she would have known that women suffered giving birth, and in reproducing generally, as a result of Eve's sinning in the Garden of Eden. While she accepted her loss as a necessary chastisement for the sake of her spiritual health, and seemed to accept it on God's terms, she also sought to know what it was that she had done wrong that she was being punished for: "I only desire of my sweet God, / The Reason why he tooke in hand his Rod? / What he doth spy? what is ye thing amisse?"

While Lucy hadn't considered God's punishment as a potential reason for her miscarriage, she also wrestled with her possible mistakes, echoing a long association between women's behaviors during pregnancy and its outcome. In the second century AD, the physician Soranus advised Roman women to avoid taking risks during the first vulnerable period of pregnancy, which he deemed to be during the first thirty to forty days when the male seed (which contained the tiny baby-to-be) could be expelled. They had to avoid an impossibly long list of potential hazards, including fright, sorrow, sudden joy, coughing, sneezing, lifting heavy weights, smelling pungent substances like garlic or onions— or anything that forces sudden movement. It makes you wonder how a pregnant Roman woman could have gone about her daily life at all.

These many strictures held fast through the centuries, and seventeenth-century midwifery manuals that circulated in Europe reflected these ancient beliefs. As the twentieth century began, things didn't look too different, and the influential American physician Dr. Joseph DeLee, often described as the "father of modern obstetrics" (also vilified for medicalizing childbirth), wrote about the threat to pregnancies from the automobile—admittedly a bumpier ride than those of today—sea bathing, sexual intercourse, hot baths, cold baths, and great mental excitements. While historical advice may seem quaint and amusing now, I frequently hear women blame their miscarriage on many mundane behaviors that could fit well in these recycled lists—such as playing tennis, eating spicy food, or even standing too close to a hot oven. In one recent study, around a third of women blamed their own actions for their loss, and I'm surprised the figure is so low.

We don't know enough about the links between certain lifestyle factors and the risk of sporadic miscarriage—or indeed how these links affect the risk of recurrent miscarriage. But it is generally accepted that women shouldn't smoke, should be of a healthy body mass index, and should limit their alcohol and caffeine intake. Recent guidance about the treatment for recurrent miscarriage suggests the same. Other identified risks include the pregnant woman being around certain toxic chemicals; taking prescribed and nonprescribed drugs; contracting listeria, toxoplasmosis, or salmonella; conceiving multiples; and being of "advanced maternal age." At thirty-five, this just about applied to Lucy, which gave her another reason to feel at fault.

Advanced maternal age (i.e., over thirty-five years) is associated with a decline in both the number and quality of eggs, and we also think advanced paternal age (over forty years) is a risk factor for recurrent miscarriage. While the risk of miscarriage in women from the age of twenty to twenty-four years is thought to be around 10 percent, it jumps up quickly to 25 percent from the ages of thirty-five to thirty-nine, and again to 51 percent in women from forty to forty-four years. Most women I talk to about their desired motherhood know full well that they shouldn't "leave it too late," but I have yet to meet one who has cracked the elusive formula that can create a sustainable relationship (if desired) and fulfill professional aspirations in the ideal fertile period of her life. Life doesn't always happen that way, yet this reality won't always prevent a woman from blaming herself nonetheless.

Historical concerns about "mental excitement" or "violent passions" have persisted in a new form, however, and emotional trauma, major life events, and stressful employment have been linked to miscarriage in some studies, though much more work needs to be done to confirm or refute these findings. The associated role that stress has on a pregnancy is a particularly thorny one: it is an amorphous concept that can easily be co-opted by women to hit themselves with, especially when no other explanation for miscarriage is on offer. Recent—confusing—advice states that "The impact of stress on the risk of miscarriage or recurrent pregnancy loss is unclear," but then goes on to state that "stress is associated with recurrent pregnancy loss, but couples should be informed that there is no evidence that stress is a direct cause of pregnancy loss." Meanwhile, the NHS website explicitly states that stress has no bearing on risk.

Research has also attempted to pursue links between stress and an inability to conceive. These studies often make their way into the popular press and popular mind, and I hear many women graft their take on these onto their experience of their miscarriage. However, according to one leading researcher in the field, Professor Jacky Boivin, researchers have yet to conclusively determine psychological factors that influence reproduction. Boivin suggests that stress has far more of an effect on the *behaviors* of people, such as their avoiding self-care, and reminds us that people reproduce in times of war, famine, and poverty. She proposes that future research should attend to what can protect us from the effects of stress, rather than trying to avoid the unavoidable.

None of this research stops women I know from worrying that their stress levels affect the health of their unborn, and it's one of the easiest factors to latch onto—not least because we can always find instances of it. One recent study showed that three-quarters of women attending a US prenatal clinic thought that a mother's stress can negatively affect a pregnancy outcome, with a third believing that pregnant women should avoid the upset of a funeral or a violent film. I look forward to more scientific and medical clarity in years to come, so that women can confidently ease up on themselves.

It may be that my own profession has played a role in the seemingly seductive reasoning of blaming pregnant women for their miscarriages and infertility. From the 1930s, psychological papers often explained women's reproductive problems by way of complex unconscious (and Freudian) conflicts that would either prevent conception or compromise the development of an embryo. Some of these papers make disturbing reading: two studies, published in the late 1960s, explore how miscarriages could be caused by a woman's unresolved psychological issues—one because of "sado-masochistic conflicts," another because of a woman's poor "feminine identification." While I don't think these particular ideas hold a tight grip on therapists' minds these days, I have heard colleagues discuss pregnancy loss through the lens of unresolved childhood wounds.

Lucy's guilt was all-pervasive, and it soon tangled up with another common—and unspoken—feeling after miscarriage: envy. It pained her to see other women's pregnancy bumps, and even to hear good news from newly expectant parents. "Every day there was a reminder of what I didn't have, and desperately wanted—a 'gender reveal' on Facebook or scan photo posted, or a pregnant bump on a magazine cover." And when her sister announced her pregnancy, the envy she felt became especially uncomfortable: "Of course I was so happy for her, and excited to be an aunt, but I was also so resentful not to be pregnant too—and this makes me feel terrible."

Lucy's envy was normal: nearly every grief I have encountered after miscarriage has included a version of this feeling at some point. But we don't tend to like being explicit about this feeling, and I haven't found any research that prises this open in any detail. The author Angus Wilson wrote, "Envy has the ugliness of a trapped rat that has gnawed its own foot in its effort to escape"—and it is, after all, one of the seven deadly sins of the Catholic tradition. But envy isn't a homogenous human phenomenon, nor does it always involve all the "ugliness of a trapped rat." While malicious envy can motivate someone to damage another, the benign type is far more concerned with motivating ourselves to get what it is that we lack—and in the context of miscarriage, this can often mean doing all that it takes to have another, live baby.

We see an extreme case of envy related to pregnancy loss played out in M. L. Stedman's tragic novel *The Light Between Oceans*. Tom is a traumatized First World War hero, hired as a lightkeeper at Janus Rock off the Western Australian coast. He falls in love with a local woman, Isabel, and after their marriage, they suffer two miscarriages in three years. Not long after their second loss, a rowboat washes up on a nearby shore containing a dead man and live baby girl. Crazed by grief, Isabel persuades Tom to pass the baby off as their own, rather than report their find to the authorities. Even this, an extreme—and fictional—example, is on the benign side of the envy divide.

I remember my own envy well. During the years of my pregnancies, it seemed that every woman I knew could get pregnant and give birth nine months later without hiccup. Their struggles to conceive and early miscarriages were often, I later learned, hidden from view and suffered in silence—making it difficult to find a community. A month after my second miscarriage, a friend invited me to her baby shower in an unusual effort to cheer me up. Furious at her lack of thought, I made an untrue excuse as to why I wouldn't go. I was genuinely delighted that her baby was on track for birth (and I delight in the fantastic teenager she has grown up to be), but I couldn't bear being up close to something I so yearned for: a baby inside me that was so likely to live. And I—briefly—hated her.

During the weeks that Lucy and I met, life events like this—baby showers, birth announcements, appointment dates—carried on as usual around her, Cass, and Freddie. A small and invisible bomb had gone off in Lucy's world, yet she quickly felt left behind in her anguish, and no one took the time, or seemingly had the inclination, to hear the full story of her second baby's short life—a life she had been able to tell me about in its complete and necessary detail. Her mood was low, and her grief unabating.

WHILE LUCY COULDN'T FIND THE opportunities she wanted to talk about her miscarriage among her social circle, she found it even more tricky to navigate conversations at work. She had never before revealed intimate details of her life to her professional world, but an early miscarriage can force us into a revelation that we may not be ready or even willing to make. We may want some people to know what has happened, but usually it is those of our choosing.

Despite discrimination laws to protect women, many women I speak to feel that their employment position can be vulnerable after disclosing a pregnancy or—in one fell swoop—a pregnancy and its ending. A miscarriage is mostly interpreted by colleagues, a manager, or an HR department as a plan to have a baby, and it follows that another pregnancy—or attempt—is in the cards: such details of our family planning are usually kept private.

While some women choose to keep their miscarriage secret from their workplace, risking "marking their card," Lucy felt otherwise. "I couldn't face lying about having time off, and I didn't want to pretend it hadn't happened." Lucy came clean and asked her manager for two weeks off—she had no way of knowing how much time she should give herself to recover. If a family member had died, she wouldn't have thought twice about taking many weeks off. If she had had a hysterectomy, she would have had at least six weeks off. She had no set of coordinates for this event though, nor did her boss have any—so two weeks was a bit of a guess. Had she gone online, she may have had guidance: women often share their recovery periods, and workplace experiences, with each other.

Lucy's manager was compassionate and easily agreed to her request (which she would treat as pregnancy related, so kept separate from her sick record), but she didn't know enough to leave it open for Lucy to extend her leave if need be or to suggest that she could come back gradually. Her return to work became another instance of the jarring relationship between her inner and outer worlds: while her job remained the same, her sense of herself had become wholly different. She was no longer the woman doing the tasks she had been doing while pregnant and infused with dreams of a maternity leave and the mothering of two. "I walked around the block a few times before I could step inside. I felt so raw and so exposed. I know I looked the same from the outside, but if you had cut me open like a stick of rock [candy], the words inside had changed."

There are very few places that are well adapted for the bereaved after a miscarriage—maybe in a labor ward or early pregnancy unit, or among some friends or family, or, most probably, in a support group. The workplace is often a particularly tricky setting for any grief to have the support it needs. As one research paper concludes, "Where the main concern is 'the bottom line' or achieving other corporate objectives, it is very easy for key issues about being human to slip to the bottom of the priority list—or even off the agenda altogether." Jobs have to be done, and people often have to be near each other to do them—including those we may not know well or even like.

"My first day back to work was horrible. I didn't know who knew what, and I didn't know whether to be honest among people who weren't my good friends." Lucy's boss did her best but also struggled with what to say or do, partly because there were no established guidelines in the organization. Ideally, she would have met Lucy soon after her return to check out how she was and what she needed—perhaps to ease in slowly, to establish boundaries of confidentiality, and to have extra support if she were to get pregnant again. But most of all, Lucy needed her boss to look her in the eye and acknowledge what had happened straight off.

LUCY'S RETURN TO WORK exhausted her further, and with some encouragement on my part, she and Cass took a week's holiday. I had no doubt that Lucy had returned to work too soon and that she needed a change of scene. She returned to meet me again looking gray and exhausted, and I worried that her mood had slipped even more. I then spotted a gleam in her eye and the edge of a smile that told me, instantly, that she was pregnant. She was, at around six weeks, already at the mercy of nausea and relentless fatigue and even had to bolt out of the room midsession to vomit in the bathroom next door. She was delighted yet deeply anxious, and still grieving for the baby she had lost.

Anxiety is the hallmark of a pregnancy after miscarriage and tends to heighten even more if miscarriages repeat. On a good day, Lucy could just about chalk up her loss to "one of those things that happen," with hope and confidence that her new pregnancy would lead to a live birth. Her physical symptoms were debilitating, but they also reassured her that she was still pregnant. But these good days were random and rare, and our sessions over the early weeks of her third pregnancy would often focus on resourcing her through her fluctuating fears.

Lucy became even more hypervigilant about her health, her activities, and any twinge she felt in her abdomen. Every time she went to the loo, she feared seeing blood, bracing herself before looking behind her into the bowl or at the toilet paper in her hand. As she had miscarried before, her hospital's early pregnancy unit offered her an early scan at eight weeks, but she decided against it: "I want to do my best to treat this pregnancy normally. But I also don't want to see the baby on the screen, in case I get too attached."

Lucy's fear of bonding with her unborn was understandable: her confidence in her body and new baby had been shattered by her loss. Her mind oscillated between two babies: the invisible one she urged to live, and another she had no physical trace of or memories that others could share. While only one lived inside her, both lived in her mind, and she couldn't find many places to talk about the two of them together: "The few people I have told are so excited about my pregnancy, they ignore my miscarriage. It's as if it has suddenly been canceled out. Of course I want to be excited, but I also don't want to pretend my second baby didn't happen."

Lucy's mood lifted a little as she progressed safely past the week she had miscarried, and even more so as she edged toward her twelve-week dating scan, when she knew that the odds of miscarriage would dramatically drop if all looked good. We began to have tentative conversations about plans for her next child, and as she had done a few months before, this touched on childcare arrangements and double strollers, and fears attached to life as a working mother of two. I knew exactly when Lucy was due to have her scan: it had been the potential sun on the horizon since the appointment had been made. When I received a text from her that day, it landed on me with a thud: "Sorry Julia,

I can't make our session tomorrow. Scan showed our baby died a week or so ago." That's all I learned that day, and when we did meet, a couple of weeks later, Lucy was still in a dreamlike state of shock.

On the day of the scan, Lucy and Cass had dropped Freddie off at his day care, arriving at their appointment with trepidation as well as some excitement. They'd gotten this far after all. But as the ultrasound wand glided over her belly, Lucy detected something in the sonographer's expression that alarmed her. "Her face slightly changed, and her silence became deafening—it felt that it went on and on. I was squeezing Cass's hand so tightly, it hurt him. I asked her more than once to tell me what was going on, but I knew what she was about to say before she said it: 'I'm sorry, but I can't find a heartbeat.' I still replay those words over and over in my head.

"The sonographer turned the screen off and told us that she needed to get a doctor. She left the room, and I wiped the gel off my belly and Cass helped me get dressed. I tried to turn the screen back on, but Cass stopped me. I just wanted to see my baby. She came back and took us to sit in the waiting room outside, where I sobbed in Cass's arms. The waiting room was full, and I felt badly for the other people seeing me so upset. But I also didn't want to see other couples delighting in their scan pictures."

Some hospitals have designated rooms for couples after they have been given bad news, and some women with healthy scan results are asked by staff to wait until they have left public waiting areas before they look at scan photos in order to protect couples like Lucy and Cass. These are important protective measures for the bereaved, and campaign work continues to push for them to be effected in more hospitals. Lucy and Cass were eventually offered the privacy they needed, but not in an ideal position: a doctor ushered them into a consulting room off the side of the waiting room. "As we went in, I remember dreading having to face the waiting room again as we came out again."

Unlike Lucy's first miscarriage, this one was referred to as a "missed" or "silent" miscarriage. She had had no idea that her baby had died, but it was probably only a few days before. As she sat down with Cass by her side, she—yet again—faced a painful discrepancy between her own needs and that of the medical system attending to her. "The doctor was kind, but she was clearly in a hurry. I remember how she didn't sit down in the chair in front of us—she remained standing, leaning her bottom against the edge of a desk. She kept pressing and releasing the tiny button on her pen as she spoke—I wanted to grab it and throw it across the room; it was difficult enough to take in anything she was saying." Hearing this, I wondered if her doctor would have clicked her pen lid while discussing the treatment of a different life-altering event, such as the removal of a limb, which is how another woman described her miscarriage to me. Maybe she would have, if it was a symptom of her own distress.

Lucy and Cass needed time for their news to sink in, to ask questions and to take in the answers. Time may also have allowed their doctor to tune into their relationship to their pregnancy more closely—to hear their use of the word "baby" and to find out what the miscarriage meant for them both. But doctors don't always have enough time in busy clinics, let alone appropriate physical spaces in which to speak to grieving couples. One specialist bereavement nurse I spoke with reflected on the indivisibility of compassionate care and time, and how the former often relies on enough of the latter. She spoke of a doctor she knew who *would* take time with a grieving and shocked couple, but this meant that other patients were left waiting, with the risk of them having to return the next day.

As a therapist, I'm spoiled with the time I have with clients—I may have multiple fifty-minute sessions and complete privacy in a comfortable room. But even if medical staff lack what I have, little shifts in their delivery of care could make a huge difference: Lucy and Cass would have appreciated their doctor sitting down, leaving her pen alone, and looking them both in their eyes while she spoke. She could have conveyed a sense that she was talking about bad news, rather than an event that needed management by medical means. And if she had been distressed herself, perhaps sharing this would have been a human, useful, feeling to share too.

The doctor gave Lucy and Cass a hospital leaflet called *Early Pregnancy Loss*, which set out what she had quickly described: the options for how Lucy's third baby could, as it would need to at some point, leave her body. There was nothing in the text about why her baby's heart had stopped beating, and as this was Lucy's second miscarriage, she wasn't eligible for tests to find out why—for now, investigations pursue "recurrent" miscarriage, which is defined after three consecutive miscarriages are endured. "Nature" seemed to have had its way again, although her body was resisting following its usual course, because her baby was still inside her.

"The leaflet said I could wait for a miscarriage to happen naturally, but there was no way of knowing exactly when my body would let go. I could also choose 'medical management,' which meant returning to the hospital to take drugs that would either start or speed things up. Or I could choose 'surgical management' under anesthetic. We were encouraged to decide before the department closed that day, so we had only a couple of hours to think things through. All I remember about our journey home is my repeatedly asking Cass whether I was still pregnant or not. I felt like a human coffin again: nothing seemed to make any sense."

Lucy couldn't bear the thought of going through the torment of another sort-of birth at home, and despite her desire to avoid medical interventions as much as possible, she opted for surgery with general anesthetic. This wasn't without its risks, albeit small: she could pick up an infection, suffer damage to her uterus, or even have to have it repeated—and repeated—if it was unsuccessful in removing all that her pregnancy had created. She would have dreaded a C-section for Freddie's birth had it come to it, having wanted to fully participate in his arrival in the world. But this time, she had no emotional strength to participate, and as much as she felt that this was the worst way that her body could part with her baby, it was also the only one she could face.

In electing surgery, Lucy also had some certainty in the midst of a lot of ambiguity and unknowns: she would know the time it would take place, and that it would be over when she woke up. "I just wanted it to end." When I had surgical management after a miscarriage in 2008, I remember feeling similarly. Back then, it was routinely called an ERPC—evacuation of retained products of conception—and while this ugly term lingers among staff in hospitals still, it has been officially replaced with a softer descriptor: SMM or surgical management of miscarriage. It may even be called a D&C (dilation and curettage), as it is in the US. Lucy would have balked at hearing "products of conception," as I did, so it was a relief to me that this didn't happen to her.

Seeing Lucy after her surgery was difficult—I am never immune to hearing about the pain a miscarriage has caused, and while I know only too well that healing takes time and support, a part of me still hopes each time that I can say something magical that can evaporate the pain. As I imagined she would, Lucy had slipped back into guilt and self-blame, but another feeling emerged that I hadn't heard from her before but echoed other narratives I've encountered. She felt she was a failure—as a wife, as a woman, as a mother and a person. "I have now lost two babies, so there must be something wrong with me. I couldn't keep them safe. I have let Cass down, my parents down and also his parents—they were all so excited, and all so wanted Freddie to have a sibling. All my friends are having their second baby now, or so it seems."

Lucy is far from alone in damning herself in this way. The baby-loss charity Tommy's ran an online survey about the experience of miscarriage in 2015—the #MisCOUR-AGE campaign—and a staggering 79 percent of the six thousand participants said that they felt like a failure, and much of this relates to a powerful cultural assumption that a woman should bear fruit. Just as Lucy had experienced after her first miscarriage, questions about her fecundity keyed into her sense that she was expected to bear more than one child. Her day could be ruined by someone innocently asking, "Is Freddie your only child?" A reasonable question of course, but one that may not always land softly on an invisible grief.

Lucy agonized over questions about the size of her family, as many women after miscarriage do. "I don't want to say the truth: that I have one child, but lost two others—especially as my babies weren't stillborn nor died after a full-term birth. There is no obvious vocabulary for them." The pregnancy loss community has talked about "angel babies" for years, but this cultural vernacular isn't really spoken elsewhere—nor does the term suit every bereaved parent. I relate to Lucy's dilemma, never knowing whether "two boys" is an honorable answer to the question of how many children I have, but I continue to hope that we can find easier ways to talk about our almost family-members, in whatever way feels right.

Neither Lucy's shock, guilt, resentment, anger, and envy nor her ongoing and oscillating grief were unusual. Just because her babies' bodies were tiny, and her pregnancies yet to be socially established, these facts had no bearing on the size of her anguish or the physical endurances she had been through to part with her much cared-for babies. Nor did the existence of her living child cancel out all that she had been through. But most of this part of her pregnancy story wasn't fully grasped by others—at work, in hospitals, and among friends—and like many women, she felt let down and isolated on top of all else.

Three

A Conspicuous Absence

LATE MISCARRIAGE

For sale: baby shoes, never worn.

—Ernest Hemingway, attributed

My first miscarriage, when I lost my twins, happened in the twenty-second week of pregnancy, which is an extremely rare occurrence. It is generally accepted that only 1 to 2 percent of all pregnancy losses concern babies who die after twelve or thirteen weeks. We tend to assume a pregnancy is safe if all goes well at the twelve-week dating scan, which detects abnormalities and measures a baby's growth, and also generally marks the time when we reveal its existence to the world—with a grainy black-and-white photo to prove it. But as I was to learn more than once, my babies weren't safe just because they had made it past the best-known hurdle: their late miscarriages, or very early births, involved greater physical onslaught and a grief compounded by their increased definition in the world.

Like its "early" counterpart, "late" miscarriage is a term

that absorbs a large range of experience: from a loss soon after the first trimester (twelve weeks) to a birth of a baby born dead at twenty-three weeks and six days—or nineteen weeks and six days in the USA. Thereafter, legally, a baby isn't miscarried, but is born "still" and must be recorded so on a legal register. Miscarried babies, as yet, have no such official record.

This demarcation between early and late miscarriage is important, partly because the factors associated with causation can differ between the two, but also because their medical treatment treads different paths. If a late miscarriage threatens, it is far more likely that a woman or couple, will turn up at the hospital for help and will then remain to be treated there. In which part of the hospital she will be treated depends upon how many weeks pregnant she is at the point of loss, staff resources, and training in each setting.

Given miscarriages after the first trimester are rare, it follows that I have met fewer women who have suffered them. The same applies to the world outside of the consulting room, making the nature of this experience a particularly misunderstood one. Emma was one of these overwhelmingly unlucky clients, and she emailed me soon after the first anniversary of her daughter Rose's death, born at nearly twenty-one weeks after a sudden and unexplained labor. A visit to Rose's grave had precipitated a disabling swell of grief that concerned her, not least because she felt she had to decide soon whether to try to get pregnant again because she was forty-one years old. She worried that she wasn't feeling strong enough to go through another pregnancy, but she also needed an opportunity to tell her story from its beginning to its ongoing end.

After meeting with Emma for the first time, I understood why her grief was still so raw a year on. She spoke with an intensity that told me of the extent of her trauma: Rose's simultaneous birth and death felt, at times, like an event of the present rather than the past. Nothing could have prepared her for either of these rites of passage, merged tragically into one, and she had never felt fully able to mourn. "People think I really should be back to my old self by now, but I'll never be that person again. No one mentions Rose; it's as if she didn't exist."

Emma's journey to become pregnant with Rose was not an easy one—it rarely is in a same-sex relationship. When Emma met her now wife Jenny, she was thirty-six and Jenny was ten years older and had a twenty-five-year-old son from a short marriage to her childhood sweetheart. When they decided to become parents after a couple of years together, Emma was the obvious candidate because she was younger, but also because she wanted to experience a pregnancy. Luckily for them both, an old friend of Emma's, Richard, agreed to be their sperm donor, and when this arrangement was finalized, the couple celebrated with a low-key wedding to affirm their commitment to creating a family together.

Trying to conceive through a home insemination kit isn't always plain sailing, and coordinating schedules around Emma's ovulation was difficult for three busy people. There was no way around the fact that the couple had to make great effort to make a pregnancy possible. Emma did her best to maximize her chances of conceiving by following fertility advice, critically aware of getting older and therefore losing reproductive time: she knew her chances of conceiving and carrying a baby to term were slipping away as the months passed. "The first few times of trying were quite fun, and Jen and I would plan a romantic evening together once Richard had left the flat. But after the first few times, it was far from fun—I became completely consumed by the process. My life revolved around chunks of two weeks: waiting to ovulate and then waiting to do a pregnancy test. My period arriving was hellish for us both."

After their seventh attempt in the course of a year, the couple struck gold. They decided to share their long-awaited news with the friends who knew about their journey to conceive. But they held back from telling work colleagues, which was relatively easy to do as neither woman experienced the same expectation to have children that heterosexual couples can. Each was wary of being sidelined in the respective academic departments they worked in. "We had both witnessed female friends lose out on opportunities the moment they announced their pregnancy. They were immediately treated as if they weren't committed anymore and not asked to collaborate on projects. So we decided to wait as long as possible."

Emma and Jen also faced another type of prejudice: from those who assumed Jen wasn't a mother too. Parenthood is still routinely thought of as a heterosexual endeavor, unless it begins in a fertility clinic that no longer thinks twice about treating same-sex couples. "At my first booking-in appointment at the [prenatal] clinic, our midwife asked me if Jen was my friend. We were holding hands and wearing wedding rings! Even after I told her that Jen was my wife, she asked who the father was, which was totally irrelevant." Jen's experience of invisible expectant motherhood is far from isolated.

Statistics about lesbian motherhood internationally are vague, but one study estimates that a third of British lesbians are mothers and another that, in 2013, around twenty thousand dependent children lived with same-sex parents in the UK. According to the 2001 Australian census, 19 percent of female same-sex couples had children, and a 2009 study in Canada published a similar figure of 16 percent. These are not insignificant statistics, yet we know little about a lesbian partner's experience of a pregnancy and even less about her experience of miscarriage. One feminist researcher, Lisa Cosgrove, writes of this in impassioned terms, noting how research agendas and conclusions are informed by assumptions about "compulsory heterosexuality," and that "the voices of single or lesbian mothers and nontraditional couples are nowhere to be found in the research literature . . . [this] must be addressed so that 'women's responses' to pregnancy loss are not conflated with 'married heterosexual women's responses' to pregnancy loss." Nearly fifteen years since her writing this, these assumptions may have loosened a little, but not nearly enough.

Emma and Jen were both nervous about the pregnancy as they had supported friends who had miscarried or had, like them, had to work extra hard through assisted conception to conceive—either because they were same-sex couples or because they were heterosexual and had faced infertility. In these, often grueling, conditions, the process of trying to conceive and the event of a subsequent miscarriage can become so intricately bound that to understand the sense of loss of the baby, one has to also consider the stressful journey it took to create it. Emma summed this up by saying, "It felt like we'd given so much blood, sweat, and heartache to get pregnant in the first place." The couple was relatively lucky too, as they hadn't had to make great effort to find a sperm donor or employ the expensive services of a fertility clinic. But however much the couple felt cautious, they would still talk from the early days of pregnancy about their baby becoming a part of their future lives. "We discussed names, talked about sabbaticals from work, and even began to think about moving home."

Emma's first trimester turned out to be blissfully uneventful, and her routine twelve-week scan showed that her baby was thriving: its crown-rump length—the standard measurement of growth—was as it should be, along with a strong beating heart. The combined results of a nuchal translucency measurement—tracking the thickness of fluid buildup at the back of the developing baby's neck—and blood test pointed toward a minimal risk of chromosomal problems. "We left the hospital that day elated. Jen wanted to post our scan picture on Facebook, but that felt too much for me—I wanted to know who knew."

I can't speak for Jen, but I wonder if her desire to share the scan photo more widely was a reflection of how her baby had become more real to her after seeing it on an ultrasound screen. She hadn't felt the physical symptoms of a pregnancy that Emma had by then: the painful breasts, nausea, fatigue, interrupted sleep, and heightened sensitivity to smells. She may have remembered her own pregnancy of course, but that was with a different baby from the one for which she was now filled with pride—and maybe love. The black-and-white image gave Jen visual proof of a baby she knew existed but had less of an inescapable and visceral connection to. Emma told me how Jen carried her scan photo around in her wallet and made its image the home screen of her phone.

As much as Emma felt more reserved about sharing the news of their baby with the wider world, it wasn't long before she had little control over who knew about her new status as a pregnant woman. A month after her scan, at around sixteen weeks of her pregnancy, Emma's belly had swollen so much, she had to buy new clothes. As had happened to me in some of my pregnancies, both her slimness and the warm weather meant that her pregnancy bump soon became obvious: "I still remember the first time someone offered me a seat on the bus to work. I enjoyed my new bigger body and that people could see my precious cargo, but I also resented how I suddenly became public property."

Emma was entering a stage of expectant motherhood that was no longer hidden from view. The more a pregnancy progresses, the greater its embodiment: both of the baby in the womb and of the pregnant body. While an unborn develops into a recognizable baby-like form that we are more comfortable with holding in mind, a pregnant body also becomes a recognizable mother-to-be too, and it's not just a swelling belly: breasts enlarge, a woman's gait changes, and skin and hair can noticeably change texture. Other people could *see* Emma was having a baby, whether she wanted them to know or not.

Being offered a seat on a bus by a stranger was a kind gesture, but Emma read other signals from the public as more judgmental. Even before she revealed her pregnancy to anyone, she responded to the many cultural messages as to how to manage her body and behaviors, and she became hypervigilant about all that she did, ate, and drank for fear of harming her unborn. Once her pregnancy became more obvious, she found that this policing became more explicit. Women have long been ripe for judgment as bearers of future children for the community, and perhaps even more so when we look—or are known to be—pregnant.

The historian Professor Laura Gowing has written about how extreme this surveillance of a pregnant body could get in a context far removed from miscarriage. She describes a time and place, in seventeenth-century England, where single women were seen as a threat to the social order—especially if they became pregnant. A woman could be closely monitored for pregnancy signs, sometimes brutally: bellies were felt without warning or, even worse, nipples squeezed for milk. This level of scrutiny is clearly horrific to the contemporary mind, and clearly exceeds what women I know endure for their pregnancies now, but today's women can still feel a stark contrast between other people's interest in both their non-pregnant bodies, and their baby who died.

Like Emma, my belly provoked other people's unsolicited interest only when it expanded—being offered a seat felt kind, but comments about my biking to work or my vegetarianism could feel less so. Emma's experiences were similarly tricky: "We were at a party a couple of weeks before I lost Rose, and I was having a small glass of champagne. Someone asked me if it was alcoholic—she knew perfectly well it was but was clearly having a dig. And then at the same party, someone else put their hand on my belly without even asking me. I seemed to magnetize people when Rose was inside me, but it was the opposite once she had gone."

As Emma's pregnancy progressed, she felt Rose move inside—barely distinguishable fluttering at first, and later more definable movements that could be felt from the outside by Jen's hand. Emma could sometimes translate what was a kick and what was a punch for Jen's mind's eye. This so-called quickening has had a vexed legal meaning through English history, and its officially sanctioned diagnosis was used as a defense in criminal law for centuries—allowing a condemned woman a reprieve from her death sentence until after the birth of her baby. "Quickening" meant the baby had a recognizable legal (and spiritual) status, and while this distinction no longer holds true among the women I talk to, a baby's movements can form indelible memories of a life later mourned—as Emma so described.

I still retain the memories of the movements of those babies that were big enough for me to feel—it's hard to describe a set of imprints in my body rather than my mind. During my first pregnancy, I would lie alone and marvel at the strange shapes being made out of my own flesh. By this stage, my internal world had become enormously enriched: my dreams were vivid and I enjoyed an increased level of introspection—the early trace of primary maternal preoccupation that the influential psychoanalyst Donald Winnicott described taking hold of mothers soon after birth. He saw that this state of being prepares a woman for motherhood by allowing her to tune in closely, and intuitively, to her infant. For me, the longer the pregnancy went on, the more opportunities existed for these reveries.

By the time Emma and Jen reached the halfway point of pregnancy, the name game they had long been playing resulted in Rose for a girl, Max for a boy. Their routine mid-pregnancy anomaly scan, when detailed measurements of the baby's body would be taken, along with a check of vital organs and developing skeleton, was booked for twenty-one weeks. Excitingly for many parents, the gender of the baby is obvious to the sonographer's trained eye at this scan too, but the couple resolved not to know: "We knew everything possible there was to know about her conception; we wanted one unknown."

They began the daunting task of clearing out their joint study to turn it into a nursery—nesting doesn't always happen in the last few weeks of pregnancy. A friend donated a Moses basket and a pile of small sheets and onesies, and another gave them hand-me-down toys and a baby monitor. Objects for Rose, and representing Rose, started to find their place. "Most of our friends had kids and we had a list of who was going to give or loan us things. We even began to think about a color for the nursery walls. Jen is a brilliant artist and she began to design a mural for the biggest wall: a woodland scene with lots of animals, birds, and magical creatures. She left a space in the design for either the word Max or Rose."

One evening a couple of days before her second scan, Emma was sitting on the floor in the nursery-to-be, sorting through piles of old papers. As she leaned forward to grab another file, she felt a gush of warm liquid rush out of her. "At first I thought my bladder had gone. I stood up to go to the bathroom to clean up, when it happened again: a small jet of straw-colored liquid burst onto the floor. I called for Jen, who immediately knew it was amniotic fluid—she had had a baby before. She called for an ambulance and got my stuff together. The paramedics were fantastic, and at that stage I thought we had a problem, and I was terrified, but I also thought that everything would be okay."

On arrival at the hospital, Emma was admitted to the labor ward, with Jen having to explain to more than one member of the staff that she was the baby's mother too. Although largely geared toward the likelihood of live births, labor wards have considered, and adapted, for the tragic event of a birth of a baby who has died or will die, more and more —with great thanks to sustained campaign work.

It was very busy that night, so the couple was led to the only empty room available—in between rooms with laboring mothers inside. Maternity units in England increasingly provide a dedicated room for a birth leading inevitably to death—separated from happier births—but it was, tragically, already in use that night. Not all that do exist are out of earshot of newborn babies' cries either, another crucial detail that continues to be campaigned for too. Unsurprisingly, some women don't want to be on a labor ward at all.

When a woman presents at the hospital having a late miscarriage, she is unlikely to be sent home—nor have I met a woman who would want to. Protocols differ as to whether a woman will be treated in a labor ward or a gynecology ward. Generally, miscarriages happening after around twenty weeks are cared for in the former, although some may admit women miscarrying much earlier, after fourteen weeks. But many women miscarrying between twelve and sixteen weeks feel they don't belong anywhere, hovering in an in-between state that is neither "early" miscarriage nor "late" miscarriage. Emma told me that she wouldn't have wanted Rose's birth to happen in a gynecology ward beside women being treated for non-pregnancy-related issues—believing it's not where babies are supposed to be born.

Staff in labor wards—as they are in early pregnancy units—*tend* to be better attuned to the experiences and needs of miscarrying women, and Emma and Jen were fortunate to benefit from this increased consideration over the years. Some midwives may have had further specialist training in pregnancy loss, as an optional—sadly not compulsory— professional development, and Sands is one charity that works hard to plug the gaps of knowledge through promoting and delivering this training to any health professional who may be involved in caring for someone bereaved. And as I write, it is soon to publish the first nationally recognized job description for a bereavement support midwife for the NHS to use, which reflects an improved commitment to the role.

Sands training includes exploring the special nature of grief in relation to pregnancies ending early, but also how best to think about, and talk to, stunned and bereft parents. The principle of informed choice for couples runs like a golden thread through this particular bereavement care, including when it comes to making memories of their baby and what happens to their baby's body. This valuable training is yet to be universally taken up within and among UK maternity units, and hospital funding will have a bearing on its delivery—just as funding has a bearing on the provision of appropriate care and support for miscarrying women at any stage of their pregnancy.

A recent small study of ten final-year student midwives' experiences of caring for the bereaved after a baby has died on a ward suggests a need for further training for the inevitable experience of pregnancy loss. One quoted reflection of a student hit me the most—"I think we are used to moving around": the stillness such an event brings about is, indeed, agonizing. One very experienced midwife I spoke with remarked on the difference between her training in the late 1970s compared to today: her training in nursing before midwifery was mandatory, which is no longer the case. She discussed how this nursing experience exposed her to the broad repertoire of human illness beyond pregnancy and birth, and in particular it taught and prepared her well for death too. For some young midwives, pregnancy loss may be as unfamiliar, and daunting, as it stubbornly remains to the nonmedical world.

In her room in the labor ward, Emma's midwife examined her and confirmed that her cervix was opening, but of course Emma hoped, and believed, that Rose could be saved. "I couldn't really take on board that Rose would die: I had felt her move earlier that day. I assumed they could stop my cervix from opening—that it could be stitched." Some time after this—for Emma, this episode was clouded in haze—a doctor came to tell her and Jen that there was nothing anyone could do to stop the inevitable birth. He was clear and he was kind, but he avoided speaking the unbearable truth: that the birth would also, inextricably, mean a death. Nor did he have an answer to the question that Emma kept asking: "Why is this happening?"

Emma will always remember the moment at which Rose's death actually sank in: "It was only when a midwife took my hand, looked me in the eye, and told me that our baby wasn't going to make it that I understood what I hadn't wanted to understand. She said she was too little to survive. She also asked me if we had a name. That meant so much." As I experienced with my midwife Mat during my first miscarriage, such honesty and compassionate care were instrumental in helping Emma and Jen through the unfolding horror, and it would last forever in both Emma's and Jen's minds.

I'll never know how much support this midwife and Emma's doctor get after a shift like this. My guess is not much. This is another area of clinical practice that reform work hopes to improve—good bereavement care has to rest on staff being well looked after too, just as my own clinical supervision allows me to do the work that I do. My supervisor—and peers—help me keep perspective, watch for burnout, and support my own distress. Even staff with years of dedicated experience in caring for the bereaved can be physically and emotionally drained by their work, and their knowledge and skills may not always offer an effective shield from the trauma and pain they are exposed to.

Emma was monitored for signs of infection and progression of her labor, and when painful contractions began, she was offered an epidural. Some women have physically painless late miscarriages, with no contractions before their cervix fully opens, but Emma welcomed her suffering. "Jen was encouraging me to have pain relief, but I wanted to feel the birth as much as I could; it felt like the least I could do for Rose. If she was going to die, I wanted to suffer too. I was her mother." Emma's courage to fully engage with her labor touched me—unlike Emma, I had desperately wanted to avoid feeling either pain or a vaginal birth when labor set in with my twins, despite being told how dangerous a cesarean section could be. We all have different ways of coping with trauma, and denial has been a reliable, and sometimes costly, one for me.

The same midwife who told Emma and Jen that Rose would not survive her birth was the first person to meet her. "Your beautiful little girl is here now. Would you like to see her?" She cut Rose's tiny umbilical cord and wrapped her in a hospital blanket before giving her to Emma—after warning the couple that her skin was darker than they may have expected, because she had yet to store fat. She left the room to find clothes small enough; many hospitals now stock these specially made garments—supplied by charities—in readiness for bodies that won't yet fit into shop-bought clothes. Emma worried about Rose's appearance, not knowing what to expect or if she'd look familiar. We tend to know only what full-term babies look like in the flesh.

Rather than putting Rose to her breast as she had hoped one day to do, Emma held her cautiously and took in the stark duality of greeting a baby who she was also saying good-bye to. "I was so nervous—I had no idea if there was going to be something wrong with how she looked. But the midwife was absolutely right: she was beautiful, and perfect. I touched her face with her tiny eyes sealed closed, and briefly pretended that she was asleep. I then peeled the blanket back to examine and take in every bit of her." Emma and Jen were left alone with Rose while she remained a little warm, and a newborn baby could be heard wailing nearby. Jen would be the only person to congratulate Emma on the birth.

UNTIL AT LEAST THE EARLY 1980S, parents were routinely prevented from either seeing or holding their baby after late miscarriages and stillbirths. This practice was partly rooted in the ridiculous idea that women couldn't really bond to a baby unless it was born full-term and alive, but also in ideas stemming from Freud's influential thoughts about maternal psychology. Freud believed having a baby was merely "fulfilling a wish" on the part of a mother, so its death could be simply remedied by having another one. Furthermore, it was thought that a mother would recover best for another pregnancy by being kept calm and therefore *not* seeing the baby that had died, and that a "healthy grief" (if allowed for at all) involved cutting all ties with her loved and lost. Sedating women in these tragic circumstances was also frequent, in a futile attempt to help a woman forget.

I spoke with a retired obstetrician who cut his teeth at the time of this paternalistic, and now seemingly cruel, medical culture. He described how he knew no differently from these protocols taught to him by his senior doctors and experienced nursing staff. An evidently compassionate man, he knows very differently now, and conceded with regret the number of years it took for things to change. He referred to the impact on his profession's thinking of the reform work from two physician-psychoanalysts in London, Emanuel Lewis and Stanford Bourne. These doctors were rattled by the practice of removing babies from their bereaved mothers without their seeing or holding them, and sought to widen the scope of compassion for women experiencing perinatal loss in general.

Bourne and Lewis wrote a series of letters and articles in journals throughout the 1970s and '80s about their concerns for maternal care after babies died at or soon after birth. In one article, Lewis encouraged his colleagues to allow women to see their babies in these circumstances, noting how this could actually *help*, rather than hinder, their mourning process. He caricatured the practice at the time with a discomfiting metaphor that he clearly abhorred—"the 'rugby pass' management of stillbirth," which referred to "the catching of a stillbirth after delivery, the quick accurate back-pass through the labour room door to someone who catches the baby and rapidly covers it and hides it from the parents and everyone."

A woman I spoke to, now in her late seventies, still grips on tightly to the glimpse of her baby she bore at around twenty-two weeks in 1967, as it left the room swaddled in the arms of a nurse. I know, and she knows, that it wasn't best for her not to see her baby, even though a nurse unforgivably described it as a "monster." To this day, she doesn't know what physical abnormality her baby had to merit this heinous description—or its gender or what happened to its body after it left the birthing room that day. She continues to mark her baby's birth—and death—each year in private reflection. She has never felt able to include others in her mourning—apart from her close family—as her baby was never able to exist in other people's minds.

This woman isn't the only parent to have been scarred by the use of the word "monster," and it has a lengthy medical lineage, explored by some historians with an interest in the subject of recorded monstrous births. The language of "monstrosity" was often used for the ambiguous false conceptions—what we now suspect were early miscarriages—described in premodern medical texts. One research paper about pregnancy loss published in 1983, which was influential in highlighting the desperate need for a change in medical culture, picked up on this stubborn association between babies with developmental problems and a perceived lack of humanity.

The paper's author, Alice Lovell, interviewed staff in four London hospitals about their management of late miscarriage, stillbirth, and neonatal death. She writes, "A junior doctor, whom I found sympathetic and sensitive to talk to, also told me that he advocates a woman seeing her dead baby: 'except the monsters . . . they're disgusting. They should be destroyed . . . wiped off the face of the earth' (Dr J)." She also observed how staff subscribed to a "pecking order" of gestational loss that considered miscarriages to be less sad than stillbirth, and stillbirth less sad than losing a baby who has lived. Many bereaved I speak to feel that this hierarchy of loss still exists today—both inside and outside of hospitals.

While the contemporary medical culture is undoubtedly a universe apart from Dr. J's egregious personal beliefs, it is worth remembering that some of his patients may be alive today, perhaps still tormented by inadequate treatment and forever wounded by dispassionate or cruel words. Nor am I convinced that all attitudes beyond the walls of hospital wards are far off Dr. J's: I regret reading some shockingly dehumanizing comments posted beneath images of a baby lost to a late miscarriage that a grieving mother had shared online. Obliterating a human identity may be one absurd way of avoiding the anomaly brought by a simultaneous death and a far too early birth, but it fails miserably to achieve its goal.

Emma and Jen were the beneficiaries of a number of necessary changes made during my lifetime to the care that miscarrying women receive in hospitals—including the profoundly important choice given to them to spend time with Rose. After letting the three of them have time alone, their midwife helped them wash Rose, and then dress her—in other words, helped the couple fulfill their natural desire to mother. They had needed this help to feel that this was both allowed and normal, especially as Rose was so tiny and fragile. Shock is disempowering, but so is being confronted with an experience that has no culturally accepted script.

Pressure from bereaved families and charities has contributed to the invaluable creation of recommended good practices for the care of miscarrying women (and their partners) in hospitals. Until fairly recently though, guidance to health professionals was unclear in regard to how much choice parents should have when it came to seeing and holding their baby—a relic of previous tussles over ideas for their best care. Although guidance only directly addresses babies born after twenty-four weeks, it has profoundly influenced care for babies like Rose and my own twins.

In 2007, the then-called National Institute for Clinical Excellence (NICE) seemed to discourage parents from interacting with their babies: "Mothers whose infants are stillborn or die soon after birth should not be routinely encouraged to see and hold the dead infant." Fearful of a culture of "taking away" returning to labor wards, campaign work led NICE to supplement this statement three years later: "this recommendation is not intended to suggest that women should not be given the choice of seeing and holding their baby, but rather that they should not be routinely encouraged to take up this choice if they do not wish to."

It is now clear that parental choice about contact with their baby is the overriding best principle of care, and those parents who decide not to see their baby should not be pressured to change their mind. But they should also be given time to talk and think about it, in case they do. Choice—as informed as it can be at a traumatic time—is crucial throughout all decision making after any miscarriage, as it keeps the power with a vulnerable parent, where it should rightfully be.

What research has been done shows that those who do see their babies lost to late miscarriage don't regret it, and Emma proved the same. She clearly treasured the time she had with Rose and the memories it allowed her to collect of her, and the couple will always be able to describe her appearance and how it felt to have her in their arms, as well as in Emma's womb. We don't yet know enough about how it is for parents to spend time with much smaller babies—the research isn't there yet—nor is it something we talk about.

I *was* pressured to meet my twins, and it upset me at the time. I was far too scared—of what they would look like, and of having to face up to what had just happened. I chose to rely on the bank of memories I had accumulated before then, including a handful of scan photos, their movements inside me, and the unforgettable experience of their staggered labor. My ongoing pangs of regret—and deep shame—could never have been predicted by anyone at the time, least of all me. But after hearing stories like Emma's, I wonder whether I would have chosen differently if someone had told me that they were beautiful or made washing them or dressing them seem like a natural thing to do. My mother did tell me much later how lovely they were, but it was too late by then.

My only experience of meeting one of my late miscarried babies was a very strange one, as a result of the trauma my brain was coping with at the time. In my sixteenth week of my fourth pregnancy, I spent a long night in accident and emergency, vomiting and cramping but without any bleeding. My attending doctor had told us that she had little experience in pregnancies under threat, nor could she track down any scanning equipment to discern whether my baby was either safe or alive. I was eventually discharged with a wishful diagnosis of gastroenteritis and a terror of yet another loss.

Moments after returning home, I felt a pressure on my cervix and rushed to the loo. Copious blood, tissue, and clots left me, but I caught my small baby as it took its slower path in their wake. I brought it up to my lap on the palm of my hand, but I didn't see anything: only a nothingness I can't put into words. Just as I had with my previous, much earlier miscarriage, I then flushed the nothingness away. Many months later—for reasons I won't ever fully understand—my mind delivered the image of my tiny, perfect-looking baby to me. My "seeing" eventually married with my lasting memory of "holding," but I'm still not sure if it helped me come to terms with my loss.

For Emma and Jen, their time with Rose allowed them to underpin the reality of her brief, largely hidden, existence in the world. They had no memories of Rose breathing or moving, or of her sounds or the smells her body could have made. But being with her in the delivery room allowed the couple to create and collect valuable memories of her, that, in turn, would also nourish their ongoing relationship with her. Emma's memories of caring for Rose became valuable "hooks" for her to think about and talk about with Jen and with me—and to the very few people who were curious to know more about her.

Ariel Levy wrote about this tragic sense of ephemerality after the death of her son, born prematurely in a hotel room at nineteen weeks: "He was not someone who slept and played; we did not have routines; he had not established preferences or facial expressions." But she goes on to impress on the reader the preciousness of the time she spent with him, not least because it provided her the opportunity to make memories to enrich her ongoing bond with him. Importantly, it also allowed her to record an instance of it: "I took a picture of my son. I worried that if I didn't I would never believe he had existed."

Emma and Jen were also able to take photos of Rose during the short time they had to parent her. I don't know if they displayed the images for others to see on the walls of their home or on Jen's Instagram feed, where curated images of Jen's son and Emma's swollen expectant belly resided with pride. I doubt it. Family photos tend to capture times that are memorable for happy reasons, while Instagram tends to favor idealized moments. A photo of a dead and very tiny baby is contradictory to what we expect to see.

I have two polaroid photos of my twin girls, taken by someone I don't know. They remain in an envelope in a box under my bed, and I keep them there so as not to disturb myself and other people—unlike Rose, my babies weren't dressed, or lying together as they should have been. They are, frankly, presented as clinical specimens, and I am heartened to know this form of photography is highly unlikely to happen today. While I hate to look at them, I treasure their concealed nature nonetheless: like Levy describes, they offer objective proof that the twins and their births actually happened.

Of course babies lost to early miscarriages can be photographed—or recorded for YouTube as Nico in my previous chapter did—but many women I speak with prefer to picture the baby that they had in mind, along with a scan photo if they had one. We protect ourselves from anything not considered normal, and visual images of early miscarried babies have yet to claim that status. They also can't be photographed if they are flushed away, and many hospital protocols encourage staff to caution women who have surgical management: removal from a womb under this procedure will damage the bodily integrity of a baby. Unfortunately, one grieving mother I spoke to was warned of "the bits and bobs" that would result from her surgery by a member of her surgical staff—words that no doubt will haunt her forevermore.

These days, many parents have smartphones to capture images of their babies, and some hospitals now offer a digital memory card to be taken away as a memory to, literally, hold on to—along with the images it can store. In the US, the charity Now I Lay Me Down to Sleep coordinates a network of volunteers who offer professional photography services to grieving families, and while this charity is growing internationally, it has yet to gain traction in the UK.

There is also a growing interest among some hospital staff to take photos for parents, and I spoke with one bereaved mother, Rachel Hayden, who now spearheads training in a particular method of specialist remembrance photography for babies lost in late miscarriage and later gestations. Rachel was taught by the US photographer Todd Hochberg, who is celebrated for his stunning documentary-style images of grief and death. She was drawn to his approach of capturing a narrative around a loss, and how this can help with the positive memory-making for a family coming to terms with their grief.

As Rachel described, this isn't about creating a technically beautiful photograph, which may be staged or arranged. She encourages staff to take many photos that capture an experience of a very precious and intimate time, without intrusion or direction by the photographer or props. This may mean other family members are included, as part of the story depicted. The photos should, in her words, be able to "provide a memory of that time that is real, unfussy, true but sensitively taken, focusing on details and emotions." Rachel acknowledges that parents can be afraid of the reactions of others if they show their photos, and she suggests to staff to also capture "easier to view" feet or hands as well, for sharing more widely.

Although we are undoubtedly in a visual age, the desire for a visual representation of a dead baby is clearly not a contemporary one. The nineteenth-century practice of postmortem photography wasn't considered odd, as death was then less hidden from our lives. One small study of a handful of sixteenth- and seventeenth-century paintings shows how wealthy families, financially able to commission portraits, recorded their very young loved and lost. Catherine de' Medici and Henry II of France memorialized their three lost infants in a private portrait produced for Catherine in 1556: it shows a small crowned boy, Louis, in front of two tightly swaddled babies—Jeanne and Victoire. We don't know at what stage of pregnancy these twins were born or when they died, but like many bereaved, perhaps Catherine took some strength from this poignant proof of their brief existence.

Emma and Jen had about half an hour with Rose to cherish and record their existence as a family together—it may even have been extended if there was a cuddle cot available

for Rose to lie in. This looks like a conventional Moses basket, but its small mattress is filled with cold water that allows
a tiny body to be preserved longer than room temperature
makes possible. Some parents choose to take their baby home
with them in this cot, to cherish more parenting time before
having to decide about what to do next. Many hospitals now
have one to hand, and charities raise funds for more to be
stocked: tragically, there may well be more than one needed
at the same time.

WHILE THERE WAS NO DOUBT in both Emma's and Jen's minds
that Rose would last forever in their joint family narrative,
Emma spoke of the concern that she would have no official
permanent record. Under UK law, a baby born dead before
the twenty-fourth week of pregnancy is the event of a
miscarriage—and there is no official recognition of this
baby. A baby born dead after this gestation is a stillbirth, and
is required to be legally registered as such. A stillbirth also
means that parents become entitled to parental leave and
other legal benefits as they would for a baby born alive. In
Italy and Spain, a miscarriage can happen until twenty-six
weeks, although the European Medicines Agency suggests
twenty-two completed weeks, and Australia and the USA
use a twenty-week boundary. But Rose was miscarried, not
stillborn, so she was neither required—nor permitted—to
be officially certified or registered.

Emma and Jen were, and are, far from alone in resent-
ing the legal situation in the UK: a number of petitions
and individuals have campaigned for a lowering of the

twenty-four-week boundary. The impassioned MP Tim Loughton is at the center of one of these efforts, and as I write, his private member's bill progresses through the many stages of becoming law (and by the time of publication, it may or may not be enacted as law). The bill includes a request for a report on whether our current law on stillbirth registration ought to be changed—either to allow the registration of pre-twenty-four-week pregnancy losses (so it is a personal choice) or to require it (so it is a legal requirement). A *Pregnancy Loss Review* project by the Department of Health & Social Care is also considering the issue of registration of pre-twenty-four-week pregnancy loss, along with a wider review of care and support for women and their partners.

Sands is concerned that any change to the current law may hamper their efforts to monitor stillbirth trends and causes and say that most parents they support agree with them. The Miscarriage Association canvassed the views of their members in an online survey: the overwhelming majority were in favor of *allowing* registration of a pre-twenty-four-week loss at any gestation (74 percent of 2,586 respondents). Less than half, 44 percent, were in favor of *requiring* registration. I think the position statement published by the charity in May 2018 strikes an appropriate note: it supports a change in the law *to give the option* of registering losses that occur before twenty-four weeks. The meaning ascribed to a miscarriage is not the same for everyone. The charity also sets out a number of conditions for its support, including a recommendation for a full national consultation and a guarantee that any proposed legal changes must have no implications for abortion rights or limits. This is a highly emotive and deeply complex issue that feels very live as I write.

After an early miscarriage, the bereaved often come up against a cultural assumption that there was no "baby" who was lost—it's a "bag of cells," "just a pregnancy," or "at least it was early." But when miscarriage happens later on in pregnancy, especially after a more familiar birth process on a labor ward, this status is less precarious in many people's minds—not least because of a baby's increased embodiment. But at the same time, a miscarried baby of whatever gestation is not *quite* a person, because our law says as much. Emma and Jen cared deeply about this lack of statutory validation for Rose: "Rose was our child, and I could see that she was to our lovely midwife too. Jen remembered the pride she had felt when she registered the birth of her son, and it hurt her deeply not being able to do the same for Rose."

In place of a certificate from a legal register, Emma and Jen were offered one created by the hospital—a simulacrum that many hospitals offer, and many parents appreciate, but which neither of them wanted. "We thought that it would remind us that Rose *wasn't* officially recognized. We can change our mind and ask the hospital at a later time—even now, a year on, I keep changing my mind; it depends on how angry or sad I feel." I was glad that this option was left open for the couple, and it made me wonder about my own feelings about such certificates (that I wasn't offered), all these years later. For many bereaved, such a long-after retrospective validation can be powerful—especially if the existence of a baby was denied, maybe even decades previously.

In the UK, until 1992, babies born dead before twenty-eight—not twenty-four—weeks of pregnancy were miscarried (reflecting that viability was different then), and very often, hospitals wouldn't keep records of these miscarriages or the means of disposal of the babies. Babies would be routinely taken away without parents being told how or where they would go next or being given any sense of a timeline. Sands now helps bereaved parents find out where their stillborn babies may have been or were buried but, along with the Miscarriage Association, can face a difficult task with a miscarriage, where there is often no paper trail left. Just as Emma and Jen were offered an endorsement of Rose's personhood by the hospital, Sands offers a bespoke "Certificate of Birth" for babies "disappeared" years ago too: a simple—yet profoundly potent—statement of existence, with a baby's name, parents' names, and date of birth.

I can't see how there will ever be an internationally unified view on when a miscarriage becomes a stillbirth, nor can I ever see this legal boundary not being of concern to parents like Emma and Jen and to researchers of pregnancy loss and stillbirths. The World Health Organization attempts to sum up a fetal death as "the intrauterine death of any conceptus at any time during pregnancy," but how this translates into legal definitions of miscarriage and stillbirth throughout the world varies enormously—as do our moral, emotional, religious, cultural, or spiritual views. Problems also arise from varying parameters used, including birth weight, body length, and/or the clinical estimate of gestational age thresholds.

If Rose been born dead in the US, she would have been

stillborn. Up until fairly recently in the US, however, only her death—rather than her birth—would have been officially recorded, by the issue of a certificate of fetal death to a parent. Many bereaved parents felt aggrieved by this painful and explicit denial of a birth, and years of campaigning work by the MISS Foundation has led to the implementation of a MISSing Angels Bill—as I write, this has been effected in thirty-four US states, with three more states pending. The bill means that bereaved parents are now granted a Certificate of Birth Resulting in Stillbirth instead.

EMMA AND JEN left the hospital without any certificate and also without Rose: this isn't supposed to happen after a birth. Both parents were determined to try and understand what had ripped their lives apart, so they agreed for her to have a postmortem, which would mean transferring her to another hospital with a specialist lab. After it was completed, Rose would be returned to her birth hospital, and her funeral arrangements would go from there. Thinking about the postmortem of a baby who you have just given birth to is almost preposterous—birth and death are not supposed to collide like this. But the brutal truth is that parents have to do so, as the best results are achieved when a decision is made soon after birth—and death.

Emma was in a daze while a member of the staff described the postmortem options to her and Jen. Staff must not skim over the details of what a perinatal pathologist can do, not least because informed consent to such procedures became a sensitive issue in the UK after scandalous practices (where no parental consent was gained for investigations and disposal) were unearthed in pathology labs in the 1990s. Rarely, a pathologist may be available at the hospital to explain the process him- or herself, but usually—not always—a member of the staff with specialist training will explain to parents what investigations can be performed: an extensive one or a limited examination, with the latter providing less potentially useful information.

Emma and Jen faced an inescapably hard choice. "It felt so wrong to let Rose's fragile but perfect body go somewhere we didn't know. But we also needed to understand why she had died—so we agreed for her to be opened up. We were reassured that her body would be respectfully treated and accompanied at all times when she was transferred from the hospital. I couldn't bear the thought of her being alone or in the dark." Emma and Jen had to remind their consent taker that Jen would be signing any form too. New recommendations suggest that at least an hour must be allocated for the process of consent taking in this context, and that parents should also be told of the likely time scales for the return of the baby.

Even experienced members of the staff can find this area of practice emotionally demanding—one perinatal pathologist interviewed for a research project spoke of her preference to *not* meet with the parents before investigating a baby. She described a need to protect herself from overwhelming emotion, poignantly adding, "Of course you remember cases. I remember all my babies, some ones more than others." Some pathologists understand and anticipate with great compassion parents' fears of leaving their baby with a stranger, in a strange place: I heard of one asking a mother what music she wanted played during her baby's procedure.

But a postmortem can fly in the face of our instinct to leave our loved ones to rest in peace—perhaps especially so when our loved one is so desperately young. A recent innovation, offered in just a few hospitals in Europe, is for a postmortem MRI (magnetic resonance imaging) scan instead. This noninvasive method of investigation—where a tiny body doesn't have to be cut open—may well help bereaved parents think about postmortems with greater ease (and meet cultural requirements where dead bodies should be left intact and complete). In turn, this option may also improve uptake rates, which could increase the amount of data for valuable research into the causes of late miscarriage and stillbirth. I'm hopeful for this to become more of an option for parents in years to come.

Although neither David nor I could face saying either hello or good-bye to the bodies of our twins, we were sure about our need for them to have postmortems. We signed our form in moments, at a time when parents generally received little explanation of what the procedure would involve. Like Emma and Jen, we needed to know *why*, but I didn't agonize in the way that Emma did, as I refused to engage with what it would involve. Our twins turned out to be the only babies of ours whose bodies could be investigated: our other babies' bodies were flushed away or, in the case of my surgically evacuated one, disappeared without trace, probably incinerated with clinical waste—a practice that has been radically reappraised. We waited many weeks for our postmortem results, and shortly before the appointment set up to discuss them with a doctor, I talked to a friend about my fears of either inconclusive or worrying results.

This friend had been attentive to my grief in the immediate wake of our loss and had sent me a lovely note of sympathy. Yet when we met a couple of months later, she voiced a jarring surprise about the postmortems that echoed other people's ignorant remarks about what had happened to me and David. She couldn't translate the swollen girth of my pregnancy into the reality of it containing two tiny humans whose bodies had then been—I still hope—carefully taken apart. Her eyes widened as I talked about the impending results, and she then asked, "How did the babies come out?" It eventually dawned on her what my late miscarriage involved.

WHEN EMMA AND JEN RETURNED HOME, waves of more grief hit hard. During their time in the hospital, Jen had texted close family and friends to keep them updated. A good friend living nearby had keys to their flat and would often feed the plants when the couple went on vacation. With the best intentions, he had removed all traces of Rose's belongings from the nursery-to-be to his own home, leaving a bunch of flowers on the kitchen table with a kind note. Emma told me how much this hurt. "I know he meant well, but I was furious. The Moses basket, the blankets, the onesies, and other stuff were more links to Rose. I felt empty enough as it was, and I needed those things near me. And I hated the flowers as they were only going to die."

Emma wanted Rose's things at home, to return to, to

join the other tangibles the couple had been given by the hospital staff in a memory box. This box held footprints and handprints of Rose, along with a set of identical clothes to the ones she had been so carefully dressed in, and other mementos. These things would become the best replacement for Rose. A bereaved father writing about his baby Matilda in an academic paper about a father's experience of stillbirth also reflects on the things his daughter left behind: "the runner-up prize to her first tooth, her kindergarten drawings, her soccer trophies, a flower from her wedding bouquet, and pictures of her children."

Along with photographs, such tangible connections to a baby can help nourish the ongoing bond a parent has with him or her, and which are a natural part of grief. They help us resist any urge to "forget"—which is what Emma felt the removal of Rose's things had conveyed, and which she also felt the world expected from her thereafter. She also needed these things to help forge the identities that she, Jen, and Rose would struggle to have in the world outside her home and labor ward—as mothers and daughter. Emma remained disconcerted: "I have nothing to show I was a mother and feel unsure about claiming the role. And 'miscarried baby' will never be a good enough description of Rose—not that anyone has asked me to describe her."

Neither Emma nor Jen was in any hurry to leave their home after their return from the hospital, however empty it felt. "I dreaded the idea of seeing other pregnant women. The couple in the flat beneath us had a newborn baby, but strangely that bothered me less. I couldn't get used to the emptiness of my body—but then a couple of days later, my milk came in. My breasts, already bearing stretchmarks, were suddenly huge and really painful. I didn't know what was going on, but Jen knew, as she'd breastfed her son."

Lactation after miscarriage usually occurs after only about sixteen weeks' gestation, although I have heard of it happening even earlier when a mother has breastfed before. It only happened to me after my first miscarriage, with no warning from the hospital, making it a complete—and unwelcome—surprise to me. Women are often not well enough informed about the possibility of their breasts filling with milk after a late miscarriage, nor of what they can do with the milk if it happens. If it is discussed, they are often prescribed medication to suppress it—but making it go away may not suit everyone.

Emma felt strongly positive about her milk from the outset: "I was making it for Rose, and it felt like I was keeping a link to her. Jen bought a hand pump—I don't know how she had the courage to even buy it—and I expressed it into some pots we had remaining from our insemination kit. It was a relief from the pain at first, but then I decided to keep it going for a while. I was thinking about Rose every waking moment anyway. And pumping milk every three hours gave me a structure to my day. We buried some with her ashes, and I still have some in the freezer."

But Emma didn't feel easy about talking with other people about keeping her milk, just as she detected an unease about talking through any of the details of her trauma: "I mentioned it to one friend on the phone but she went quiet—she clearly thought it was odd. No one asked how my mind was falling apart, let alone anything about how my body was coping." I

understand why Emma felt isolated. We tend to avoid thinking about the details of bodily fluids and tissues that are lost
during or after miscarriages, especially those encountered at
home, alone and racked in grief, fear, and shock. And it's not
just the visceral experiences of pregnancy loss that remain
hidden and hushed, icky and yuck: menstruation, all traumatic births, and menopause are avoided topics too.

Donating milk after pregnancy loss is a relatively new
possibility for women and is not yet routinely suggested in
the UK—although I'm delighted to see support for this idea
in new recommendations for practice. Human milk banks
most usually collect donated milk from mothers of live babies to nurture other premature or ill babies in hospitals, or
to mothers who can't nurse their babies themselves. At the
time of writing, the UK has sixteen regulated human milk
banks, the USA twenty-two, and while these banks' policies
around donation after a late miscarriage may vary, I hear
that women are also finding ways to give their milk away
through online communities. This modern form of wet-
nursing can be a valuable resource for bereaved mothers, as
well as for the babies who are receiving the milk.

A newspaper in Philadelphia reported the moving story
of how one mother, Amy, used donation to cope with losing
her son at twenty weeks. Having been told that she wouldn't
lactate as her pregnancy loss was too early, she was unpre-
pared when her milk did come in, and began to express, at
first, to release her discomfort, just as Emma did. She movingly described her reasons for continuing, remembering a
calmness it gave her, but also "a powerful closeness to my
Bryson . . . Pumping milk in Bryson's memory felt so very

right. All life has meaning, and my son's life was no different. I decided to embrace his life's purpose."

Amy researched how she could donate her milk, and continued to pump for eight months, producing ninety-two gallons for vulnerable babies: an astounding act of commitment and compassion. After my son was born at twenty-eight weeks, he spent three months in a neonatal unit, feeding from my expressed milk, so I know how exhausting, painful, and effortful this can be. I also know that some may wonder if Amy's efforts prolonged or worsened her grief, but her reported words state otherwise, and my experience tells me that women tend to know how best to make sense of their loss.

I felt differently to both Amy and Emma when my milk came in after the twins' births. In the same way I couldn't face many realities of that time, I also resisted my breast milk because it was a reminder of the babies who wouldn't be there to suckle—and of the body that had let me down. Following my mother's advice, David bound my breasts to make it stop. If any leaked out, I washed it away, just as I did with my tears and my blood. Ariel Levy, writing in her memoir about the late miscarriage of her son, likens her milk to a bleeding from her pain too. It was only many weeks later that I felt proud that my body did what a mother's body was programmed to do: in one sense I hadn't failed after all.

AS EMMA SAT WITH ME months after she had expressed her milk for the last time, she battled to make the space in her mind and heart for another potential baby. I knew that her grief had been compounded by her and Jen's isolation: while Rose would always be a part of their lives, the fact that she had left so little a mark on others was often the toughest part to bear. No one had asked to see photos of Rose or to find out if she had been buried somewhere, or even how the couple had spent their time in the hospital together: all of this was for Emma and Jen alone. And a year on, when we first met, Emma felt an anger at Rose's invisibility, a yearning for her presence, and the tug of a tenacious guilt.

As is the case with most miscarriages, Emma's sense of responsibility for what had happened was heightened by the lack of reason given for what had caused Rose's early death. The predictably long wait for the postmortem results yielded no concrete answer for the couple. "We were told that there was a sign of infection in the placenta, but no one could know if this resulted from my cervix opening up—or whether my cervix opened up due to an infection. There wasn't much to say, and the doctor steered the conversation toward our next pregnancy. However hard he tried to assure me otherwise, I still wonder what I did wrong."

Late miscarriages are more likely to be investigated and to be given a cause than earlier miscarriages, although this cause may not be watertight. And many investigations are only able to rule out causes, without offering another. Some known causes of late miscarriage can also cause earlier losses—such as antiphospholipid syndrome (or Hughes syndrome: a disorder of the immune system that causes an increased risk of blood clots)—while others may be those given for stillbirths too. The baby may have had chromosomal problems (such as Down syndrome) or genetic problems or a problem with his or her developing body, such as spina bifida or a heart defect. If a woman has an unusually shaped womb or weak cervix, either of these may be a relevant finding too, along with infections affecting her baby or amniotic fluid. Like countless others, Emma and Jen remain hopeful that future research will provide more specific answers.

Emma's varied and ongoing feelings about her miscarriage were not wholly different from those of the women I speak with, like Lucy and Claire in previous chapters, who miscarry in their early weeks of pregnancy. But the increased promise of Rose's safe arrival in the world, with Emma's surer role as an expectant mother meant that it was afforded different clinical treatment from an early loss—as well as being of a greater shock to all involved. The couples' experience of parenting Rose in the hospital—albeit briefly— underscored what is little known outside of its walls: that she existed outside of Emma's prominent belly as well.

Four

Again and Again and Again

RECURRENT MISCARRIAGE

Prolonged endurance tames the bold.

—Lord Byron, *Mazeppa*

Just as no miscarriage can ever be the same as another, neither can the experience of what comes in its wake. Every pregnancy, and each abrupt ending, is embedded in its own constellation of circumstance. But when a miscarriage follows a miscarriage, or miscarriages follow a miscarriage, the forbearance of repeated loss can become acutely trying. Recurrent miscarriage is a reproductive experience of its own, deeply unpleasant, order. When I think of any of the stories I know about couples enduring this private hell, I am reminded of both our potentially consuming and agonizing desire to conceive and the indefatigable resilience of the human spirit.

Advances in technology and medicine have given us sophisticated pregnancy tests, 4-D scans, genetic testing of embryos, and even the ability to perform surgery on a baby in the womb, but we still don't know enough about why miscarriages happen or what can prevent them. Women, and couples, can feel enormously let down, and angered, by not knowing what causes their babies to die, and increasingly marooned by a world seemingly backing away from their plight. Recurrent miscarriage (RM) can demand so much from a woman's emotional and physical reserves that her mental health may suffer gravely. When life goes on hold while the repeated cycle of pregnancy and loss takes over, it's no wonder that women, and couples, suffer anxiety, depression, loneliness, and an all-consuming despair. Of course partners suffer too, independently of the woman who miscarried, although we know lamentably less about their anguish.

RM is not only a particularly pernicious experience to live through but also it refers to a clinical description for the occurrence of three or more consecutive miscarriages. While I wouldn't wish this horror on my worst enemy, perversely, it does bring with it some advantage: eligibility for a referral to a specialist clinic (which may be in another hospital), for investigations, and, perhaps, for treatment for one of the few known causes. A guideline published by the European Society of Human Reproduction and Embryology in November 2017 suggest this definition should now refer to *two* or more miscarriages, and that they need not be consecutive (as does the American Society for Reproductive Medicine)—but at the time of writing, we are yet to know how, or if, this will affect standard UK practice.

In the UK, some clinics do accept referrals from women

who have suffered "only" two miscarriages consecutively—such as when a woman is of advanced maternal age or has known fertility issues—but I also hear of some women, and couples, who can go through more than three shortened pregnancies before a referral for further investigations may even be discussed by a doctor. National data isn't available, but I've never met a couple who didn't have a few months' wait for their initial appointment to a specialist (NHS) clinic, which may also be a long distance from their home.

While sporadic miscarriage is deemed, clinically, likely to be caused by chance chromosomal error, RM is seen to be more likely to be due to something else—hence the clinical value of investigations. RM is set apart from the one-off, or two-off, type of sporadic miscarriage—as both Claire and Lucy, from the two previous chapters, experienced. It is statistically rare—affecting approximately 1 to 3 percent of couples who attempt to build a family—but it is numerically significant nonetheless.

Investigations give only so much hope. Research seeks to improve this bleak landscape for desperate couples, but the wait for more answers is an unavoidably long one, as research enquiries can take years to complete. As it stands, less than half of couples who go through tests will be given a reason for their miscarriages—and often this cause is elusive or a result of more than one factor. There is often no effective treatment or therapy that can be offered to help either. In one study, one-third of women referred to a Danish RM clinic did not go on to have a live birth. Then again, many couples do have their dreams made true through treatment—or through sheer staggering perseverance—and there is a strong belief, although no firm data to prove it yet, that the chance of a live birth may increase as a result of elusively defined "supportive care" that the staff in a clinic setting have the potential to offer. But like stress, supportive care is something that is easy to spot but has yet to be defined for clinical purposes.

WHEN I FIRST MET CARLA, she had, after her third miscarriage, carried a pregnancy to term and given birth to her daughter, Ella, one year previously. While she said she wanted to work on an ongoing and debilitating sense of worthlessness that her miscarriages had unleashed, she had also yet to truly believe that she was a mother of a child who was actually alive. Her anxieties for Ella's health could spike so highly that she would sometimes wake in the middle of the night to check Ella was breathing, and she still struggled to be parted from her for long.

Carla had lost three babies in about the same time usually meant for a full-term gestation, so it made sense that she was extremely vigilant about losing another. But Carla's patchy support during her darkest hours and her intense feelings of isolation from those around her had left their legacy too. After Ella was born, people no longer kept their quiet distance from her, but Carla still felt aggrieved that they hadn't understood what she and her husband, Robert, had been through—Ella's arrival hadn't canceled out all that had gone before. So there was another powerful reason Carla came to see me apart from her anxiety and low self-worth: she needed a place to let off steam.

Carla's first miscarriage happened in the seventh week of her pregnancy, and she described her then-sanguine response as naive. Not all miscarriages hit hard, and some women, like Carla, make sense of their first pregnancy ending too early as a purging of bad luck, which then paves the way for a following pregnancy's inevitable happy ending. "Of course I was really sad and I cried for a few days, but I also felt that we'd gotten it out of the way. It happened quickly at home one weekend, and yes it hurt, but the pain was bearable. We were both convinced that my next pregnancy would be okay, and we focused on getting pregnant again."

The couple was lucky to conceive again after three months. The memory and upset of her only pregnancy and its abrupt ending may well have loomed larger for Carla if it had taken many months more to get pregnant again. Carla's optimism was boosted after her pregnancy ticked off more and more days beyond her seventh week, and she began to increasingly enjoy the presence of her imagined baby. After her first meeting with a midwife, she told close friends and family about her happy news and began to narrow down the choices of names. But in her tenth week of pregnancy, not long after booking the day off work for her twelve-week scan, she started to bleed.

Miscarriages don't discriminate: they can happen while shopping, cooking, sleeping, swimming, or at work. My third began moments before I stepped into my consulting room to talk with a traumatized client—I couldn't not appear, or so I thought at the time. Carla's second miscarriage also began at work, shortly before a presentation she was due to deliver. "I was feeling nervous about the presentation, and my stomach was hurting, so I thought it was nerves. But when I went to the toilet, I saw blood on the paper, and I knew that it was happening again. Everything drained out of me. I could barely stand up."

Carla had to rally, and she called Robert, who advised her to phone her doctor. "My usual doctor was on leave, but I was put through to a locum doctor I had never met. He heard my concerns, and then said he would refer me to my nearest early pregnancy unit for an assessment as soon as possible. It's a blur now, but I won't ever forget one thing he said. He said he couldn't find my notes on his computer system, and then asked me if I had had a 'proper' pregnancy before. I couldn't believe my ears."

It didn't surprise me to hear this curiously phrased question from a doctor. In all my years of hearing miscarriage stories, I have heard many clunky, clumsy, inappropriate, and even hurtful things said to a woman by a medical professional during or after miscarriage. For those who go through more than one miscarriage, the chance of this happening will arguably increase. I am sure that there has never been any malice intended, and there is also untold compassion among many staff, but injudicious words and phrases speak of a lamentable lack of training in the experience of early pregnancy loss.

I can't account for the sloppy use of the word "proper" by Carla's locum doctor, but I like to think that he grabbed it with a medical protocol in mind (such as thinking about a referral), rather than because of a medical arrogance about her reproductive abilities. It's not good enough though, which is why campaign work targets sensitive communication, and

why the Miscarriage Association has devised their own training for health professionals to think more deeply about the
language they use to describe pregnancies under threat. Lis-
tening closely, and thinking closely about language to use,
may seem like obvious pointers for doctors to take on board
when presented with miscarriage—but not so when they
have been primed to respond to it as a minor complication of
pregnancy.

Carla described how she returned to her desk "like a ro-
bot" and then made the presentation she had long prepared
for. She had nothing to soak up her blood but toilet paper,
and there was no one to talk to in the office about the
havoc unfolding in her body and mind. No one knew she
was pregnant or that she'd been pregnant before. While it
amazed me to learn she was able to perform in front of colleagues, stories of miscarriages frequently remind me of
how courageous and resourceful women can be. As soon as
she could, she made an excuse to leave work, and collapsed
into tears in the cab that took her home.

After a night of more bleeding, cramps, and no sleep,
Carla went with Robert to the early pregnancy unit for her
ultrasound scan, as arranged by the locum doctor. EPUs'
specialism in early pregnancy assessment and surveillance
means that they tend to be a better place for an early miscarriage to be thought about and talked about than in other
medical settings. Unlike doctors' surgeries or accident and
emergency, they also have specific resources to hand, such as
scanning equipment and blood-testing facilities. One guesstimate by a doctor I spoke with is that half of the women
seen at an EPU will miscarry, and the commonest reason

women show up in the first place is because a miscarriage is threatened.

The nurse who scanned Carla knew better than to leave any silence hanging in a room that was fraught with so much fear. There was no question in this nurse's mind that this pregnancy was a "proper" one. As Carla lay, unavoidably undignified, on the rough paper sheet of the plastic scanning-room bed, the nurse explained to the couple what she was seeing on the screen in front of her: a small pregnancy sac, cocooning a tiny baby who had no heartbeat. The couple's baby had died, probably a few days before. Nearly two years after the event, Carla still held on to the compassion of the immediate condolence they then received: "The nurse took my hand, looked me in the eye, and told me how sorry she was. She said the same to Robert too. It's all that we needed right then."

Carla's kindly nurse turned out to be the only emotional support she was offered that day. Few EPUs have counseling services to refer their patients to, and the unit Carla attended did not; even if this is the case, it is often a wait of weeks if not months to get an appointment. Some women have suffered a second miscarriage—or even another—by the time they can attend their first counseling appointment. Campaign work consistently flags the need for increased funding for better support for loss after pregnancy and, indeed, pregnancy after a previous loss. In the meantime, women continue to rely on the support offered by charities or stretch themselves to pay for private therapy—as they often do with me.

Carla was far from sanguine about her second miscar-riage—she was utterly devastated. She took a week off work for a "gastric illness" and barely left her bed, remembering with me the beginnings of what became the worst period of her life: "I didn't know I could actually feel so miserable or cry so much." As she grieved for the baby she had spent so much time with in her mind, and rode waves of anger at the injustice of the odds being against her again, she also described her surprise at another layer of anguish that emerged. She had no idea how much grief she had harbored for her first miscarriage after all: losing her second baby painfully awakened this. This isn't unusual, and I have met many women who find themselves grieving for previously unfussed-over pregnancy losses after a subsequent loss.

Carla and Robert told the people who knew about her pregnancy of its ending. They needed to know, and the couple hoped for their time and support. But Carla felt let down by a general lack of interest—a few cursory "I'm sorrys"— and her sister-in-law was the first of a few people to get it, unwittingly, very wrong: "At least you lost it early on again; it was clearly nature's way." Just as Carla held on to the words of the locum doctor, this comment also stuck fast in her mind, and her indignation was still alive when she spoke with me: "How could 'at least' anything be of any consolation? And how could 'nature's way' make it okay in any way?"

CARLA'S DISBELIEF, hurt, and anger in response to this unintentionally painful commiseration is sadly familiar: one of the most common complaints I hear women make after miscarriage, and miscarriages, concerns the minimizing or inappropriate condolences that come their way. Or indeed, the noncondolences too. There is a depressing universality to the pile of unhelpful stock phrases that are said: "Keep on trying and you'll get there" or "It was obviously not meant to be" or, another that Carla resented, "At least you can get pregnant easily." I prefer any words over no words, but Carla preferred none rather than ones that landed on her as thoughtless. We'll continue to struggle to get it right with words, unless and until we can bear to think more deeply about an experience we are loath to confront up close. I hope *The Brink of Being* will help with this.

In 2017, the Miscarriage Association tackled the issue of language head-on, with its "Simply Say" campaign. The charity suggests what I take for granted: it's safe to assume that a miscarriage mattered, and at the very least needs to be acknowledged: "Lost for words when someone close has a miscarriage? Simply Say . . . I'm sorry." And in my experience, it's amazing what the power of these two words, said with meaning, can have—as Carla and Robert experienced in the EPU scanning room that day. And there's often more to say after "I'm sorry"—we only need to find out what that could be.

But just as our words can often fail to adequately express sympathy and empathy, we may also need to help the bereaved to effectively convey their experience—through giving them time and a compassionate curiosity about what happened to them. Words can shackle us all, as Nietzsche wrote: "Compared with music, all communication by words is shameless; words dilute and brutalise; words depersonalise; words make the uncommon common." Carla described to me this frustration at not being able to sum up the complexity of her second loss to her sister-in-law and others: "'I lost a baby' wasn't right. I had lost a past and a future, my innocence, my unquestioned faith in my body. I had also lost lots of blood and many days of work. But I had also lost another baby before that, always tucked behind my first."

DESPITE SUGGESTIONS from friends and family to take it easy for a bit, Carla and Robert didn't wait long before trying to conceive again. There used to be a received medical wisdom that couples should delay by a few months trying to conceive after a miscarriage, but this is no longer the case, and couples are advised to try as soon as they feel ready. In fact, recent research shows that pregnancies conceived in the first six months after a miscarriage were less likely to result in another miscarriage (or subsequent preterm birth) than those conceived any later—although, as is often the case in this mysterious field, we're not yet clear why that may be.

While the grief for their two lost babies continued to haunt them both, Carla and Robert still desperately wanted to have a child, and the hope of another pregnancy offered a focus for the couple in the mire of their heartache. They lost interest in seeing friends, not least because very few were prepared to talk to them about their ongoing sadness and their fears that even more sadness could follow. When Carla discovered she was pregnant again, just a couple of months later, it was far from a cause for excitement like it had been before. "For the first time, I did the pregnancy test alone, without Robert. I dreaded looking at the result, as either way, I knew I was going to be upset. I wanted a baby more than I wanted to be pregnant." This turned out to be the third time Carla was pregnant in half a year: this is not the usual order of things.

Pregnancy after miscarriage isn't easy but pregnancy after miscarriages can often be even more tortuous. There are two tricky waiting periods: one to find out if you have conceived again, maybe with an ambivalence like the one that Carla describes, and a second to see if a pregnancy has established itself on safer ground. Waiting periods for medical investigations of serious health problems have been studied precisely because they can be particularly stressful to bear, and it is wisely thought that psychological interventions could be devised to ease this. Research has explored how these times are experienced by patients in the context of waiting for genetic screening results or breast cancer diagnoses, patients waiting for gastrointestinal endoscopy investigations, and— of greater relevance to RM—the waiting period between embryo transfer and pregnancy test during an IVF procedure. These studies show how the not-knowing of the result adds great fuel to the discomfort, which makes perfect sense to me: not-knowing in all sorts of contexts is an existential fear that brings many of my clients to therapy in the first place. After a history of RM, all that a woman or couple wants and needs to know is if *this* pregnancy will be the one to manifest her dreams.

This time, Carla preferred to think that she wasn't *quite* having a baby: this child in mind was quickly banished if discovered to be running around free in her thoughts. Her third pregnancy became a tentative one: she imagined herself in the illogical scenario of being a little bit pregnant, and this kept her in an exhausting bind. "I was trying so hard to think that I was having a pregnancy, rather than a baby. But it was impossible really, not least because all I could think about was keeping the pregnancy safe from harm. And it was the only thing I wanted in my life—I would have traded anything for that baby to be born alive and well."

Carla was far from alone in struggling to embrace her third pregnancy, and the waiting period it involved: many women who become pregnant after miscarriage or miscarriages describe a conscious desire to hold back their feelings of hope and excitement, and may even resist thoughts of a future with a separate baby in tow. Allowing for the detailed imaginings of another child becomes inextricably bound up with fears of its loss and all the heartache that follows: optimism can become quickly soaked in anxiety, despair briefly lifted by glimmers of hope.

In trying to protect her pregnancy from any possible harm, Carla's usual low level of superstition rose in a way she had never experienced before, which often happens when miscarriage repeats. She became unusually hypervigilant about all that she ate and drank ("I even washed lettuce leaves in Evian water") and she defied her own usual rationality by making regular trips to a wishing well near her office, as well as wearing a subtle fertility belt under her shirt, made from moonstone, unakite, and jade, beaded together and sold online "to align the reproductive system physically, emotionally, and cosmically."

Looking back at these actions, Carla described herself as

"going a bit crazy," but leaning toward a magical realm in these circumstances is exquisitely human, and so common among women I talk to. I too tried anything to secure what became my final pregnancy: I carried an amethyst stone bracelet in my pocket and hung an imposing African fertility mask on my bedroom wall. While I didn't believe either would help me carry a baby to term, I was also so desperate that I was open to the possibility that they might. The practice of appeasing the fertility gods may continue to be a popular one until reproductive science can answer many more of our burning questions.

Written evidence shows that early medicine—as well as cultural superstitions—took problems in pregnancies seriously in premodern days. John Hall, a seventeenth-century medic and William Shakespeare's son-in-law, was reported to have treated a female patient after a series of early miscarriages. He gave her sage to strengthen her womb, along with a treatment of crushed garnets and pearls mixed with an undercooked egg. He also advised her to apply a plaster made from turpentine and other drugs to "the Loins, *Os Sacrum*, and the bottom of the Belly" too—not so far away in idea from Carla's fertility belt.

In Hall's day, "excessive passions"—such as anger, fear, and sorrow—were deemed risky to the unborn too. But the influence of a woman's state of mind was also thought to go further than this. The now curious idea of maternal impressions can be traced back to Roman times; it implied that any "disordered" thoughts and sensations experienced by a pregnant woman could somehow be conveyed to and impressed on her developing baby. So, for example, a craving for strawberries might result in a red birthmark, while more dangerous thoughts could even cause great abnormalities.

However ridiculous this idea now sounds, I sometimes hear women talk about a belief in a different version of maternal impression after suffering repeated miscarriage, such is their desperation to ensure a healthy pregnancy. Carla was one of them: she worried that her mind could actually *cause* her baby's death. "If I found myself believing my baby would live, I worried I'd 'jinx' things. But if I didn't think about the baby at all, I also worried that it would feel unwanted and may die too."

These efforts to keep a pregnancy both present and at bay are mentally and emotionally exhausting. Carla found this difficult to cope with and she described how withdrawn, tearful, and irritable she became. She dreaded going out in public for fear of seeing a pregnancy bump and turned away from supermarket aisles that sold diapers and baby accessories. She felt she had nothing to say of interest to others, so turned down invitations to go out. Her world rapidly shrank, and her life became suspended. A vicious cycle emerged: as she shut herself away, she became increasingly consumed with her precarious pregnant state, and thus more and more vulnerable. For Carla and Robert, this lasted weeks and weeks—for others, this cycle can last for months or even years.

There is currently research—the results of which have yet to be published at the time of writing—into the use of a brilliantly simple means of support that can be given to women (in RM clinics, but arguably elsewhere too) during the waiting period for a pregnancy to establish itself after twelve weeks. In the study, women were given a small card with ten "positive reappraisal" statements that aimed to encourage positive thinking about aspects of the dire situation they were in—such as the strength gained from a kindness from a friend or a partner. They were instructed to read the card at least twice a day.

Knowing nothing about the results, my hunch is that this humble intervention could help women cope enormously—not least because other research proves similar interventions in medical practice can help to reduce stress during the wait for other life-changing results. But this card also represents ongoing care from whoever dispenses it and something concrete to hold and to do at a time when powerlessness, helplessness, and a fear to hope can free-fall together, as Carla experienced.

The potential benefit from this almost cost-free intervention seems huge, as are the cost-free interventions we can all make, outside of clinics, to support women like Carla through her distress. Looking back, Carla could see how much she needed reminding of her life outside of her hazardous pregnant status—such as her passion for film, literature, and good friendship.

WHAT TENDS TO happen for women like Carla is that no one buoys them along. We run out of things to say when one miscarriage follows another, and we may even project our own fears of another onto them too. Carla remembered this well: "When I told friends I was pregnant again, no one was enthusiastic. My mother physically stiffened—she couldn't understand why I wanted to get pregnant again so quickly. I did feel I was going crazy at times, but all I needed was understanding. Mother's Day was really difficult—neither she nor anyone else remembered the babies we had lost or the one we were rooting for inside of me."

I strongly identified with Carla's feelings: after my final miscarriage, a couple of friends bypassed condolences completely, and gently suggested that I should call it a day on the pregnancy front. And I had only had four miscarriages. When I trained to be a telephone support volunteer for the Miscarriage Association, one of my fellow trainees had had fourteen pregnancies, nine of which had miscarried. I have also heard of women suffering fourteen miscarriages. *Fourteen*. She spoke openly about how the years of pregnancies— she also had five living children—had consumed every aspect of her life. Part of this was the obvious distress of her repeated and coalescing grief and despair, but it was also to do with the tapering understanding that she got from people around her. Not only did condolences evaporate but also people seemed to convey to her that each pregnancy mattered less than the one before.

This diminishing response to repeated miscarriages reminds me of how some historians have interpreted family relationships in our past, when infant mortality rates were extremely high. By one estimate, in 1800 43 percent of the world's newborns died before their fifth birthday. By 1960, this figure had significantly dropped, to 18.5 percent, and by 2015 to 4.3 percent: ten times less than two hundred years ago. It's not outlandish to assume from these facts that our ancestors may have braced themselves for the worst to happen after birth—just as women like Carla can do in the early stages of a pregnancy, before the prospect of a full-term birth even happens. Some have assumed that parents resisted bonding with their unborn and young infants, on the basis that their survival was not assured.

Lawrence Stone is one historian who asserts that this was probably the case in early modern England: "the omnipres-ence of death coloured affective relations at all levels of soci-ety, by reducing the amount of emotional capital available for prudent investment in any single individual, especially in such ephemeral creatures as infants." He speculated that parents would hold back from both their feelings and their care of vulnerable infants, which, in turn, contributed to their chance of dying—noting the practice of wet-nursing (where babies were given to other women to breastfeed) as one example of aloof care. The psychiatrist Colin Murray Parkes, one of our leading thinkers on grief, seems to agree; he quotes Montaigne, who wrote in 1580, "I have lost two or three children in their infancy, not without regret, but without great sorrow." Other researchers quote from letters and diaries that speak of a similar indifference to miscar-riage at this time of high infant mortality.

The idea that we can become almost immune to the death of a loved one, by virtue of its probable inevitability, is one I'm unconvinced by. I suspect our ancestors battled, like Carla, with a complex range of feelings tied up with a fluctuating set of hopes and fears, and love. And after all, we can only interpret from the surviving written records, which reflect just a part of a much bigger story; the records of the inner experiences of women in our past are on the whole woefully absent.

The historian Linda Pollock has written about pregnancies of privileged European and British women in the sixteenth and seventeenth centuries and is one skeptical academic voice. She notes that pregnancies were a matter of rejoicing but also fraught with fears like the ones Carla experienced: "pregnancy was viewed through the prism of miscarriage: as a difficult, uncomfortable, and potentially dangerous condition which, unless tended with care, was destined to end prematurely." These women, like Carla, demonstrated a clear emotional investment toward their unborn and also took on a mortal risk to bear children—it was likely that they would know of someone who had died in childbirth, and it drove some wealthy women to prepare their wills in advance. Like Pollock, I imagine these frightened women's emotional responses to their unborn and infants were far more nuanced than simply indifference or a hardened heart.

CARLA'S THIRD PREGNANCY was in the grip of such psychological warfare that this made it progress at a glacial pace. "I went through the motions at work, and I was just scraping through my tasks, getting the minimum achieved. I'd come home and wait to go to bed, ticking off another day. It felt like I was on another world, looking in." No one checked in with her as her endless days and weeks progressed, perhaps fearing her withdrawal signaled a desire to be alone. But if they had swerved caution and been there to listen and understand, they could also have been there when things went wrong yet again.

Carla described her third miscarriage as particularly cruel for dashing the highest of her hopes, as it happened later than before, in her eleventh week of pregnancy. "I'd just begun to believe things may, just may, be okay." She was so attuned to her body's subtle variations that she had called the early pregnancy unit before bleeding warned her of the worst. With Robert by her side, and a different nurse from the one before, a scan revealed that her third baby had stopped growing a couple of weeks before. "I knew the drill by then. I wanted to go home and let my body say good-bye. And I suppose I had a scrap of good luck, because my womb emptied everything soon after—I didn't need medication or surgery to get rid of everything or endless scans."

Carla remembered well how she could both believe and not believe what had happened—her physical and emotional shock matched the devastation that descended. Her mood plummeted to an unprecedented low, and she battled for her mind to quiet enough at night to allow her to sleep. She feared sharing the news to those who knew about her trials, as she suspected a repeat of the lack of support she'd had before. This third miscarriage evoked another powerful dimension of anxiety too: "It hit me hard that I might never become a mother after all—or at least a mother to a living child."

Many women worry about never becoming a mother after having one miscarriage, but a reiteration of loss can heighten this to an all-consuming fear. A powerful desire for parenthood fuels the astounding strength women and couples muster in order to repeatedly conceive—or not conceive—and to bear pregnancies that cause so much heartache. And while there is no doubt in my mind about a genuine, primal yearning for a family that leads to its fruition being pursued at such high cost, I'm also critically aware of how the motherhood ideal weighs heavily in the background of our lives. Women are still expected to become mothers—and then to mother in particular ways.

In my teens, in the mid-eighties, I first became aware of the feminists who challenged the tenacious link between motherhood and femininity. Raised as a Catholic, I unthinkingly absorbed the "Madonna and child" iconography and message and as a child did not question my destined role to further my family fold. But in my late teens, the critiques of Ann Oakley and Adrienne Rich made me think about motherhood in a new, less limiting way. Sadly, Rich's powerful assessment that "the non-mothering woman is seen as deviant" still rings true, forty years after she wrote it. The authors of one recent study in Australia note how "motherhood has predominantly been perceived as natural for women, the desire for it inevitable, unquestioned and central to the constructions of normal femininity."

We live in a culture that judges those without children pejoratively—whether they choose to be "child free" or mourn their status as "childless." Men also suffer from this pressure to be a parent, but given that women are expected to shape their lives around nurturing children, they tend to feel it even more. The words littering fertility discourse don't help either: "failure to conceive," "failed pregnancy," "hostile cervical mucus," and—as my own reproductive shortcoming has been repeatedly described as having—an "incompetent cervix." These terms are slowly fading, but they are still here, and as long as pregnancies go "wrong," women will feel they are "wrong" too.

In the UK, these corrosive pronatal ideas reared their ugly heads during the Conservative leadership contest in 2016 when MP Andrea Leadsom suggested that as a mother of three, she had "a very real stake" in Britain's future, giving her the edge over Prime Minister Theresa May, who does not have any children. The abuse the former Australian prime minister Julia Gillard had to put up with from her political opposition for not having children is even more depressing. One example of scores of recorded insults shows how: "I mean anyone who chooses to remain deliberately barren . . . they've got no idea what life's about" (Senator Bill Hefferman, *The Bulletin*, May 2007).

I spoke with the author Jody Day, whose first book, *Living the Life Unexpected: 12 Weeks to Your Plan B for a Meaningful and Fulfilling Future Without Children*, became an Amazon bestseller in twenty-four hours. Her burgeoning organization Gateway Women offers an online community of support for those facing life without children: its reach is now around 2 million people. We talked about the lingering archetypes that continue to describe a childless woman: "spinster," "crazy cat lady," "hag," "witch," and even "selfish," and Jody observed, "Even 'career woman' implies that a career is prioritized over family in a counterfeminine way. I have yet to hear of a value-free English word that describes a childless woman."

Jody sees pronatalism everywhere too: "Just walk into a supermarket and you will see an extraordinary display of pregnancy and motherhood on the magazine shelves." We both remarked on the recently splashed images of Beyoncé's twin-pregnancy body. "This glorification of motherhood in the media began with Demi Moore's pregnancy bump in 1991. That was pivotal and marked a change—I'm not sure if we have reached a peak or whether there is more to come." The day after we spoke, a naked and heavily pregnant Serena Williams graced the same magazine cover as Moore did. She looks gorgeous, but I know I would never leave that image lying around my waiting room.

Jody also remarked on the powerful combination in the West of pronatal pressures with an overwhelmingly consumerist culture. We seem trapped in a need to produce and consume in order to succeed in life, with the lifestyle and material things that can prove this to each other: the home, the car, the clothes, and the digital devices. Through this cultural lens, the production of a baby becomes an integral part of this successful lifestyle, and the pursuit of motherhood thus becomes one of achievement—or, if not done right, or not at all, failing. Jody concludes that "to be fully adult means being a parent, and a fear of childlessness is codified into us."

My own profession—at least historically—isn't blameless when it comes to prizing motherhood over non-motherhood. In Freud's theories, a girl's desire for a baby was seen as developmentally normal: if she didn't want one, this suggested that things had gone psychologically awry. Other influential thinkers in Freud's wake teased out nuances of this, although ultimately they agreed that women's main developmental goal was to bear fruit. Erik Erikson, a developmental psychologist who coined the term "identity crisis," wrote that a woman has "a valuable inside, an inside on which depends her fulfilment as an organism, a person, and as a role-bearer." I'm not convinced, from conversations that I've had, that these views have entirely evaporated in the therapeutic field today.

THE EARLY PREGNANCY UNIT WAS, a few months down the line, still lacking in resources for the ongoing emotional support that Carla needed after her third miscarriage, and she had little hope of accessing it through her regular doctor either. Pregnancy loss isn't singled out for poor emotional support—as a therapist, I know only too well how dire provision is for many mental health problems. But Carla had never felt so badly before. "I couldn't sleep, but I couldn't get out of bed either. After a week, I went to the doctor to sign me off work for much longer, but I had to go through everything again, with another locum doctor. She used words that made little sense to me—she asked if I'd had a 'blighted ovum,' or if I'd passed all the 'pregnancy tissue.' She didn't use the word 'baby' once."

Our spoken medical vocabulary is derived from its written scientific language—and in the context of miscarriage, there are many words that can miserably fail to capture a woman's understanding of her body, her baby's body, and the fraught processes that separate the two. This language continues to evolve, but not comprehensively or universally yet, and words do leak out that disturb and hurt—"fetal demise" or "hydatidiform mole" can't ever describe the death of a yearned-for baby.

I still can't shake off one particular verbal exchange. After my miscarriage at around sixteen weeks of pregnancy, I lay on a hard plastic bed with my knees bent and my heels near my bottom, while a harried doctor examined my cervix and assessed the state of my womb. She ignored my tears and David's equally obvious distress. While David did his best to soothe me, a paper sheet did its best to absorb my blood as it steadily made a large ragged shape around me: as miscarriages are prone to do, this one had rendered me completely vulnerable. Even though hospitals were familiar to me by then, I was far from used to being at the behest of "medical expertise," and no more used to my body taking medical precedence over my tormented mind.

Turning away from my shocked gaze and holding a gray cardboard dish in her hand, my doctor told me that I had to wait further for "the products of conception to be fully expelled," and then left the room. I literally didn't understand what she meant—it seemed that my womb was producing things *other than* a baby. She was a doctor, after all, and clearly knew best. Centuries ago, it was thought women *could* produce "products" from their wombs, such as gristle or fruit; one German doctor wrote in 1788 that "not everything that comes from the birth parts of a woman is a human being." A little earlier, in 1726, Mary Toft, of Godalming, England, managed to convince the royal surgeon that she had given birth to animal parts and rabbits, before being rumbled as a fraud and imprisoned. While I wasn't worried that I had conceived something nonhuman, I was genuinely fearful of what I was waiting for—and I understand how my ancestors may have also feared what came out of them too.

Medical language responds to the context of its time; in the nineteenth century "drapetomania" (deriving from the Ancient Greek for "a runaway madness") was the name for the mental illness that caused slaves to run away from captivity. And for many centuries, "abortion" could also mean "miscarriage" in the modern sense of the word, and the two words were used interchangeably in premodern medical works, such as Jane Sharp's *The Midwives Book*, of 1671. While "abortion" has now evolved to mean an induced pregnancy termination, it's only really since the late 1980s that doctors consciously began using the term "miscarriage" instead of "abortion" or "spontaneous abortion." A woman experiencing repeated miscarriages, like Carla and me, may well have earned the label "habitual aborter" before this change. In the UK, it was partly thanks to Professor Richard Beard, then professor of obstetrics at St. Mary's Hospital, London, that these descriptors of pregnancies cut short began to adapt to the times.

Beard, responding to his own understanding of women's experiences of loss, wrote an emotive letter to the medical journal *The Lancet* in 1985: "It is curious that, in a language as descriptively rich as English, no clear distinction is made between a spontaneous and an induced expulsion of the contents of the uterus in early pregnancy." As ugly as some of his latter words may be, his letter was hugely influential and I'm grateful for it anyway. He also noted how a contemporary survey by the Miscarriage Association showed that 85 percent of women who had had a miscarriage wanted to change the word "abortion" in the context of spontaneous loss. Like me, he recognized the "unmitigated misery," "fortitude," and "deep disappointment" of miscarrying women, as well as their "uncomplaining" nature while "at their lowest ebb."

Thanks to Beard's plea, practice began to change, at least in written journals. At the start of the 1980s the *British Journal of Obstetrics and Gynaecology* used "abortion" for miscarriage in every instance, while by the end of the decade, not at all. However, "spontaneous abortion" still lingers in international research journals and in Spanish *"aborto espontáneo /natural"* refers to miscarriage, which can sometimes lose nuance in translation. A recent survey in the US showed that 88 percent of respondents preferred the terms "miscarriage" or "early pregnancy loss" to any other words. Those who preferred "spontaneous abortion" or "early pregnancy failure" were more likely to have had an unplanned pregnancy or a previous history of a planned abortion.

I know I'm not alone in disliking the word "miscarriage"— it persists in its connotation of its original meaning of "error or mistake," with its unavoidable finger-pointing at the once-pregnant woman. One researcher consciously writes about "involuntary pregnancy loss" or "IPL" in her paper; more recent research refers to "early pregnancy loss," and the most recent clinical guidelines on the treatment of recurrent miscarriage refer to "recurrent pregnancy loss" too—so maybe this heralds a move toward a different label. Although many feel that "loss" can imply a forgetfulness or a carelessness—or, ironically, something mislaid.

AS WELL AS her use of jarring words, Carla's brief appointment with her doctor rattled her for another reason. "She asked if I wanted to take antidepressants. She was already typing out the prescription before I had even answered her. I didn't need a prescription! I just needed someone to listen to me and understand what I was feeling." As Carla watched the doctor type, she felt that only parts of her story had been heard, the insomniac and depressed part, which meant that the other parts of her story—the enormity of her losses, pernicious sense of worthlessness, and fears of never being a mother—had rapidly vanished away.

I'm not against medication to treat symptoms of acute mental distress. But I also know of the healing nature of empathy, compassion, and understanding as a first step to addressing the potential deep anguish after miscarriages. While the doctor endorsed her time off work with a sick note, Carla clearly needed counseling or other further support to help her bear the unbearable. It may well be that there were no psychological services Carla could be referred to (these are thin on the ground), but her doctor didn't think to discuss private resources or point her in the direction of charities that aim to plug this enormous gap.

As Carla spoke of her disappointing and—not unsurprising to me—cursory appointment, I thought of how different this seemed from the medical encounters described by the physician Dr. Johann Storch in eighteenth-century Germany, analyzed by the medical historian Barbara Duden in her book *The Woman Beneath the Skin*. Dr. Storch kept extraordinarily detailed accounts of his consultations with his middle-class female patients, including pregnant ones, that provide us with a fascinating insight into the depth of interest he had in, and importance he attached to, a woman's vivid description of her inner sensations and bodily processes. It seemed that he *really listened* and worked hard to be guided by his patients, rather than jump to a ready diagnosis.

Of course, Storch had the time that modern overworked doctors don't, and he had little else to rely on but his patients' narratives—no technology or permission to examine these female bodies. But when I read about his close attention to the detail of a woman's narrative, I was struck by how miscarrying women today lament their opposite experience. They often report hurried medical encounters and how priority is frequently given to their physical rather than mental health. And while they may be happy to be a patient, they also want to be treated as a patient in such holistic terms.

Carla's doctor spotted that she was perhaps depressed—which is potentially a good thing of course—but Carla felt this was too swift a judgment and that it bypassed a proper assessment of her distress. The nature of her profound grief, and the rupture of the future it involved, had been rapidly glossed over. But in contrast to Carla, many women also experience mental health problems after miscarriage, or miscarriages, that are not picked up on at all, or at best discounted as normal.

Ever since the research community began to take miscarriage more seriously, studies have sought to measure its psychological consequences: grief of course, but also depression, anxiety, and post-traumatic stress disorder. There is a lack of consistency in the approach of all these studies: differing variables and profiles of participants make it hard to synchronize results, and very few studies have explicitly addressed the effects of repeated miscarriages—as opposed to sporadic miscarriages—on women in terms of mental health. We need greater clarity, so that women and their partners can be offered better treatment.

While I'm unsure how we can confidently untangle these emotional states from one another—say grief from anxiety, or depression from grief—the research does amount to what I know: the experience of miscarriage can lead to a profound distress that many people may not have imagined. It may cause a state of being that can't simply be gotten over in time, and a bereaved may need support above that given by friends and family or other usual networks. And as Carla described, when miscarriages repeat, the emotional fallout can have an overwhelmingly negative influence on all aspects of daily functioning—just as any depressive episode or serious anxiety disorder might too.

In the research community at least, it is now accepted that miscarriage can cause a profound grief, and attempts have been made to capture its intensity so that it can be taken more seriously. However, there is far more research to be done in refining how this grief is moderated or intensified—including a better understanding of how repeated miscarriage can affect a woman and her partner. Interestingly, research papers repeatedly muse on the particular nature of miscarriage grief, with its emphasis on a set of complex losses and future dreams, without ever defining it explicitly. The concept remains epistemologically immature, miserably echoing how the grief of miscarriage has yet to be fully established in lay terms too.

Varying instruments such as the Perinatal Grief Scale, Miscarriage Grief Inventory, Perinatal Grief Intensity Scale, Perinatal Bereavement Grief Scale, and Impact of Miscarriage Scale have all been used to measure grief responses after miscarriage—such as the yearning, sadness, and painful memories of loss. They all seem to point in the same direction: grief after miscarriage can be equal to the grief that follows other significant losses, such as the death of a recognized family member. These research findings have yet to trickle through to most of us though: miscarriage remains at the bottom of the pecking order of other griefs. There's some agreement among researchers that the acute phase of grief tends to abate after about six months, leveling off after a year—but this healing process has little chance of survival when one miscarriage follows another, or another, or another. Here, a grief coalesces with the next grief and the next, while contending with other relentless states too: anxiety, low mood or depression, anger, guilt, envy, and despair.

Studies exploring anxiety and depression after miscarriage are similarly difficult to pull together neatly. Some research suggests that a significant proportion of women who have recently experienced a miscarriage meet the criteria for clinically recognized depression (27 percent) and anxiety (28 to 41 percent), but that both these states tend to lessen over time, with anxiety generally lingering more. This tapering of distress is unlikely to happen when more miscarriages happen though; if anything, I see the opposite playing out with my clients. One recent Danish study of women being treated in their national recurrent miscarriage clinic highlights a significant risk of increase in stress and depression—but, as ever, it also highlights the need for further research.

Most people I know wouldn't think miscarriage could cause post-traumatic stress disorder (PTSD), but one recent piece of preliminary research points toward this, and I have also suspected this has happened for some of my clients—although I often find out much later on. This study, based in a busy early pregnancy unit, found that 39 percent of participants met the clinical definition of moderate-to-severe PTSD three months after their loss (which included ectopic pregnancies, which not all studies do).

We tend to associate PTSD with living through the horrors of war (as once called shell shock), rape, or a natural disaster. But given that it can develop in response to experiencing a real or perceived threat of death or injury to oneself or others, it makes sense that some women could suffer it after miscarriage or miscarriages. Not only do women live through the death of their baby in the closest terms possible, but they can also fear for their own physical health, or even life, such as when serious blood loss, repeated surgeries, or an ectopic pregnancy occurs.

PTSD has a number of debilitating anxiety-related symptoms, but one particularly pernicious one is of the unwanted intrusion of vivid memories that can propel a mind back to the time of the trauma—as if it's being replayed in real time. I have worked with many women who can find their minds lose control to particularly terrifying aspects of their miscarriage, and for years I was plagued by the visceral memories of lifeless baby bodies leaving mine. These memories—with sounds and smells and tiny details—would creep up from behind me to stop me in my tracks, but I was fortunate enough to have a therapist who helped me put these episodes back into the past—their rightful place.

IRONICALLY, Carla's poor mental health proved strangely fruitful. Her insomnia helped her find a source of support that would become the most valuable one she would get: online. Virtual communities for women who have suffered miscarriage may be one of the most significant shifts in miscarriage support in my adult lifetime—a second wave after the face-to-face support groups that grew up either side of the Atlantic in the 1970s and 1980s, alongside the emergence of campaign work and the foundation of our oldest pregnancy loss charities. These communities are testament to what women lack from elsewhere, but also serve as a reminder of what others could easily offer too—online or in person. And while online support can be enormously beneficial for women after any miscarriage, it can become especially so when the reiteration of loss can both shrink and freeze their lives: others going through similar experiences can often be the ones to get it best.

One sleepless night, and not for the first time, Carla went online to research the question no one could answer for her: "Why do I keep miscarrying?" The couple now had a referral to a specialist clinic, but she had at least three months to wait before being seen, and no available funds to access a private clinic sooner. Carla still remembered the first time she stumbled across an online forum: "I spent ages reading postings of things that I wanted to say but had no one who seemed to want to hear. Women were being honest about their fears, anger, and loneliness, their envy of other women who sailed through their pregnancies, and of how much they missed the babies they had lost. My friends didn't understand any of this, and I couldn't bother Robert in the middle of the night. I felt a weight lift from my shoulders that night."

Carla found a readily available place to go when she felt lonely in her grief or when she wanted to ask a question about her miscarriages, including the grueling physical and emotional recovery. With so much not-knowing, she came to rely on the pooling of knowledge and advice that other women offered, with the guarantee of being heard too. The reciprocity of grief, despair, hope, support, and compassion was hard to find elsewhere, and she ascribed the improvement in her mental health to the community of support she found there. Her mood slowly lifted, and she began to sleep better and, above all, feel less painfully alone. She didn't take her prescribed antidepressants.

The moderators of the two Miscarriage Association Facebook forums tell me something similar: women (because members are almost exclusively women) seem to fill the gaps left by the outside world, and the community of reciprocity can count for so much. They talk about their blood loss and pains, about their sex lives, the flux of their bodies and minds, as well as emotional states that they describe to have been banished or ignored in the nonvirtual world. They vent about poor or insensitive encounters with others and seek advice: about options for managing their miscarriage, about treatment for RM, and about how best to cope when the pain bites hard. It is particularly moving to read the shared commemorations for lost—often named—babies, thought about on due dates they never made, or on the twelve-week marker they were supposed to be revealed to the world.

Online communities aren't utopian by any means, and conflicts and trolling exist in miscarriage support threads as they do elsewhere, but the relative ease with which women online seem to talk about their reproductive losses doesn't yet exist in our culture in open conversation. We may whisper or use euphemisms—even women among women—yet online, bar the occasional "TMI" warning, there's a freedom I regret we don't have elsewhere. But there may be other cultures where a safe place for discussion of miscarriage exists in the real rather than virtual world, and one example can be found in the writings of Kathryn March, an American feminist anthropologist whose fieldwork among the Tamang people of Nepal in the 1980s depicts a place far removed from our networked world.

March writes about how Tamang women speak of their reproductive lives with ease: "Ask a Tamang woman how many children she has and she will answer accounting not just for her living children, but for all the miscarriages, still-births, and other deaths in between." She also observed a great deal of empathy in the wider Tamang community for these women—among the men and older generations too. Unlike Carla and other countless grieving women online,

Tamang women aren't stranded with only each other for candid talk and reliable support. The grief of lost mother-hood was *normal* and a part of the fabric of life, which of course it is.

These Tamang women seemed to have readily available support groups to help metabolize their feelings about their losses, whereas the women I talk to often have to intention-ally create them with each other, because they can't find ade-quate support elsewhere. Face-to-face groups have dwindled since the advent of online forums, but they are another in-strumental source of support for many. One group, founded by the Miscarriage Association in 2005, gets together in a hospital meeting room in central London one evening a month, and I was invited to attend by a devoted volunteer facilitator, Erin, who, when we met, had been running the group, with another volunteer, for nearly six years.

Erin told me that while some women (as it is mostly women who join) come just the once, others come intermit-tently for months if not years. I know from other groups that women can show up maybe decades after a loss, perhaps emboldened by a story in the media or by their adult child speaking up about a miscarriage in a way that was prohib-ited to them years before. Most of the participants in Erin's group have experienced repeated miscarriages, along with the increasing anguish, despair, and loneliness these can involve.

Just as happens online, a space like this may be the only container of empathy and understanding for a life set on hold. Particular dates can also provoke a need to reach out: anniversaries of losses, or due dates never made, Mother's

Day and Christmastime. One unusually big group formed after the birth of Prince George: the English media had little room for other news that week. Having a baby was made to look so easy that day, an apparently blissful and inevitable relationship milestone for a couple to enjoy.

In the group that Erin helped to run (she has since set up a group elsewhere), the hour begins with sharing stories— each participant taking a turn to describe the tiny lives that had come, and then gone, in their bodies but not their hearts. Just as I do in my consulting room, I heard hopes and fears of future pregnancies, tensions between a status as a patient and that of a bereaved mother-to-be, and the description of feelings that were difficult to air elsewhere: the pain of losing an invisible baby that may have lived more in mind than body, as well as the resentments, anger, or even hatred toward those who misunderstood or discounted what miscarriage could take a woman, or couple, through.

Friendships had been tested, family relationships strained—and in one case, a relationship had fallen apart. I detected a palpable relief among kindred spirits as the conversation picked up a pace that hour: in hearing "me too" or "that's like what happened to me." There was the valuable experience of being attentively heard, taken seriously, and empathized with—something anyone can offer, without having been through a miscarriage. This wasn't group therapy, but it was undoubtedly therapeutic. Linda Layne writes of her own experience attending support groups over the years of her seminal research into pregnancy loss. She notes her "most enduring memory" of sitting with so much "cumulative, raw, tangible pain." I was struck—but not surprised—to read that it eventually caught up with her so that she preferred to work alone.

BY THE TIME she found her valuable network of compassion online, Carla was still waiting to be referred to a specialist RM clinic so investigations could begin. Through her support network online, she gathered tips about questions to ask at her first appointment and information about research trials at clinics that might be recruiting participants to test out treatments. But mostly, her online friends made the waiting more bearable and they fully understood the not knowing if she'd ever be a mother.

RM becomes eligible for investigation because it is deemed more likely than not to be caused by something other than chance chromosomal error (which is thought to account for around half of sporadic one-off miscarriages). While we know that a number of factors may play a part in pregnancies that end sporadically, far more research needs to be done to tighten up this thinking, so that women can be confidently guided. And there is much more to further understand the mechanisms behind why a woman may *repeatedly* miscarry.

So far, we know that the older a woman is, the greater the risk of her miscarrying, and that the risk of further miscarriage increases after each successive one. Chromosomal abnormality (known as a balanced translocation) in one of the partners may be at play (in about 2 to 5 percent of couples), or a woman's blood-clotting condition may be the cause—such as antiphospholipid syndrome (the most important and treatable cause, accounting for 15 percent of women investigated for RM), or thrombophilia. A weakened cervix may explain repeated miscarriages of a later gestation too.

Treatment is on offer for APS and other clotting problems, uterine abnormalities, and cervical weakness—but none of these guarantee the outcome every couple wants. Meanwhile, research is underway to pursue other ideas around causation—such as looking into immune system responses during pregnancy, the role of the womb lining behavior during pregnancy, maternal diabetes and thyroid problems, maternal polycystic ovary syndrome, and the effect of infections.

Once a woman becomes a patient of a specialist clinic, she will consent to tests to screen for these few known complicating factors. NHS clinics tend to follow similar lines of investigation, and guidance from the European Society of Human Reproduction and Embryology (ESHRE) in late 2017 may have an effect on how and when they are made. At the time of writing, she may have a scan or more invasive investigations to detect a womb abnormality, and blood tests to detect clotting issues or role of infection. If she gets pregnant and miscarries again while under such specialist care, it may be suggested that she bring her miscarried baby into a clinic if its genetic testing is deemed clinically useful: handing over your baby to science, in a desperate effort to make another one that lives, isn't always an easy thing to do.

Many women I speak with turn to private clinics in an effort to speed up the otherwise inevitable wait for specialist care. They may borrow money, use up all savings, or even, in one case I know, remortgage the house both to free up funds for the fees and also to give up work in order to focus on conceiving and carrying a baby to term. Anecdotally, I hear of doctors prescribing treatments yet to be officially approved of by the scientific community or even disagreed with by another doctor. This can make it especially confusing and frustrating for couples who find this out.

Results can take weeks and weeks to return, and a life on hold takes on a whole new layer of meaning: more stressful waiting periods, appointment times to juggle (and maybe lie about) around work commitments, more reasons to hope—and then despair about. These clinics can become another medical arena where women can feel both grateful for help yet simultaneously objects of a disappointing science—reduced to results expressed in numbers and percentages, normal or not. One client memorably described to me how she felt her identity became her date of birth—the question asked of her each time she called her clinic. But the most excruciating and common experience is for couples to be left none the wiser, as more than half won't be given a concrete cause.

CARLA ENDED UP avoiding any investigations, as her fourth pregnancy, conceived quickly again, ended in the birth of her daughter, Ella—and no one will ever know why this pregnancy went to term. I like to think that Carla's support network may have played a part in Ella's ultimate safe arrival in the world, with its reliable compassion and consistent understanding helping to antidote the enormous threats she felt she was under: of her body failing, of another miscarriage, of friendships dissipating, and of never being a mother. We have yet to fully understand how compassion, care, empathy, and understanding affect a pregnant body under the duress of recurrent loss, but what we do have is one fascinating and painfully thin strand of research that hints toward a hypothesis.

Thirty-five years ago, a study concluded that "supportive care" (which has yet to be officially defined) in a RM clinic could in itself reduce the chance of a further miscarriage and has since been supported by others. Over a decade later, another large study showed "the excellent outcome of pregnancy after unexplained recurrent first trimester miscarriage that can be achieved in a dedicated clinic with supportive care alone." Here, supportive care referred to weekly scans of a pregnancy until twelve weeks. The authors conceded that while the evidence that this was a genuine phenomenon was very good, the mechanisms explaining it were unclear. They also conceded that such intensive management of patients would be both time-consuming and expensive, which are barriers stubbornly remaining for many RM clinics today.

Both the new ESHRE guidelines and the UK's Royal College of Obstetricians and Gynaecologists concur with the beneficial potential of treating a patient's emotional world as well as her body. The latter states in its guidelines to doctors that "Women with unexplained recurrent miscarriage have an excellent prognosis for future pregnancy outcome without pharmacological intervention if offered supportive care alone in the setting of a dedicated early pregnancy assessment unit." The guidelines of the UK's Association of Early Pregnancy Units say that staff members should be trained in the emotional aspects of early pregnancy loss, and to offer bereavement counseling. But despite this professional championing, "supportive care" remains an ill-defined and under-researched notion, which means it can't develop into a uniform treatment protocol—nor can why it seems to work be better understood.

Some studies refer to "relaxation tapes" being given to women, or the admittance to the hospital at the same gestation of a previous miscarriage. More recently, researchers in the Netherlands aimed to pin down what supportive care in an RM clinic setting could mean for the women being treated by finding out what it was that they actually wanted. Participants stated a desire to make a plan of care with one specialist doctor who knew their obstetric history. No woman I have met likes to repeat her history of pregnancies cut short, unless it's done in a spirit of compassionate inquiry. They also wanted to be taken seriously—to be listened to, and to feel empathized with—and to receive clear information about their treatment and results, as well as regular scans to offer some sense of control over the status of their pregnancy. As echoed in plenty of other research, these women also wanted specialist emotional support after miscarriage, especially if another were to happen again.

Unless and until RM clinics pursue these ideas further, perhaps through their own research and practice, and are able to dedicate resources (in both time and money) for whatever emotional support they devise for women and couples, the bereaved are likely to continue to turn to each other for support instead. We can step in too: by taking time to hear what a woman is going through, to learn and reflect on what her repeated miscarriages means for her and her partner, or even by distracting her with kind gestures—in other words, by being what a good friend can be.

In their work about the silencing of maternal grief, the academics Deborah Davidson and Helena Stahls, who are also bereaved mothers, write about the need to offer support- ive care in lyrical terms, involving "walking with them in their grief." They quote from the *New York Times* bestseller *When Elephants Weep*, in which the authors, Jeffrey Mous- saieff Masson and Susan McCarthy, observe the mourning behaviors of elephants: "A park warden reported coming across a herd with a female carrying a small calf several days dead, which she placed on the ground whenever she ate or drank: she traveled very slowly and the rest of the elephants waited for her. . . . [P]erhaps one has to believe that they be- haved this way just because they *loved* their grieving friend who loved her dead baby, and wanted to support her."

We don't yet know if any of these ideas for lay efforts of kindness and care could amount to a clinically defined no- tion of supportive care—with its correlation of increasing the risk of a live birth after a pregnancy. I can't yet know if my work in my consulting room—with its consistency, cu- riosity, empathy, validation, and understanding—may help a woman to conceive and carry a pregnancy to term. Defin- able links between our psychological health and our physio- logical mechanisms are frustratingly mysterious for many clinicians in a number of health contexts, but many of us have a hunch they exist.

The potential for a miscarriage to overwhelm and devastate is always there, but when a woman suffers the repeated experience of an already precarious-feeling pregnancy failing to thrive, a consolidating grief—in the face of little medical help, and waning emotional help—can make her even more susceptible to mental ill-health, loneliness, and despair. None of us can extinguish the consuming nature of a life stuck on hold, but we may well be able to ease it—even just a little bit—by a better understanding of what it involves.

Five

Ripples

PARTNERS, FAMILY MEMBERS, OTHERS

Would I be here if your other babies lived?

—My youngest son, aged 7, 2017

While we can easily misjudge, misunderstand, or even avoid a woman's experience of her miscarriage—or miscarriages—we also forget that the loss of a pregnancy may impact a wider range of other people too. A once-pregnant woman is likely to have significant people in her life who invested in her new status, such as parents, siblings, or other children. And there's usually one other person witnessing and participating in a pregnancy up close—the woman's partner, who is also a parent-to-be. This can make for a two-fold heartache for others when a pregnancy ends: that for the miscarrying woman, but also an individual grief for the loss of a baby whom they had been harboring dreams for and forging a bond with too.

Given the inescapably physical experience that a pregnancy—and its ending—involves, it's no wonder, and entirely appropriate, that the woman who experienced both is considered first by others, especially if a miscarriage involves medical intervention. The fact that a miscarriage happens in a woman's body contributes to why we can forget a partner's perspective, and we rarely consider that it may also have caused a family bereavement. Male partners—and as my earlier story about Emma and Jen shows, even more so with female or non-gender-conforming partners—have largely been written out of the pregnancy loss stories that we do know of culturally or been written in as an appendage or, even worse, parenthetically.

OUR CULTURAL IGNORANCE of the potentially broader emotional and psychological impact of miscarriage is reflected by the relatively small amount of research existing on a male partner's experience. What studies do tell us is that men suffer an equally nuanced and as complex grief as their partners, but that it may look different from hers. In turn, this makes male grief prone to be misjudged, minimized, or deemed as absent entirely—maybe even by his partner herself. Women who have suffered a miscarriage can feel estranged from a partner who may seem not to get it, and while of course this may well be true, many men do get it, but in their own way and often at a different pace.

Our struggle to understand the male response to miscarriage sits in a context of confused contemporary ideas in the West around masculinity and reproduction. Despite an evolution of the role of fatherhood in recent decades, into a more traditionally feminine and involved one, this has failed to usher in a safe place for men to air their vulnerabilities—which includes grief and the grief of miscarriage. Men can still succumb to a cultural expectation to feel and to express their feelings in particular ways (not too openly emotional), and to adopt prescribed roles.

When it comes to miscarriage, these ready-made roles for a man may be to support and protect his partner and loved ones, to "act" and "do," including telling others of bad news and making practical arrangements, as well as physically supporting a woman if she is left shaken, weakened, or unwell. He may want to do all of this, and it may be appropriate in the circumstances, but the net result can be that a partner's distress may not be noticed, and his actions wrongly interpreted as a signal of being okay.

Each time my body let go of my—our—pregnancies, David had to call on emotional reserves he didn't know he had. While the promise of a child evaporated for him while I called out in pain, or heavily bled, or saw no heartbeat on a screen, his desperate desire to soothe, buoy, and help me undoubtedly contributed to his inclination to swallow most of his own upset, and research shows that many men do the same.

Of course, just as some women aren't upset by their miscarriages, there are male partners who feel so estranged from the pregnancy they helped to create that their sense of loss when it ends can feel far less acute than their partner's. I have spoken to many men who dwell on the physical separation between themselves, their pregnant partners, and their growing babies—especially in the early weeks, when a miscarriage is most likely to happen and which is before they have had a chance to see their baby on a scan or feel kicks through a swollen belly. Some struggle with their truth—and concurrent guilt—that their baby was too abstract for them to mourn.

Jon Cohen, the author of *Coming to Term*, which explores the history of research into miscarriage, describes in the book his struggle to identify with his wife's pregnant—and then miscarrying—body. There's no doubt about the emotional turmoil Cohen went through during their four miscarriages, not least because it clearly propelled him to pursue his tireless research. But in reflecting on his wife's wave of intense grief on the due date of their first baby, miscarried at six weeks, he writes: "I know more intimately than anyone else what miscarriage meant to Shannon. But from another vantage, any woman who has miscarried has a more precise understanding of Shannon's sense of loss. A woman lives through a miscarriage. A man, no matter how devoted, only observes it." But even if a man does only observe, as Cohen asserts, miscarriage can be a deeply distressing observation to have to make.

While I talk to many men in my consulting room (although, in general, I have far fewer male clients than women), I hardly ever talk to them about miscarriage. Nor did I speak to many men when I volunteered for the Miscarriage Association as a telephone supporter. Those I do meet tend to do so at the arrangement of their partner—either with her or, more rarely, alone. I met with Cass because his wife, my client Lucy (featured in my chapter about early miscarriage), had encouraged him to see me and had liaised with me to set up his appointment. It's rare for me to see both of a couple separately, but Lucy was convinced he needed a space to speak freely and that he wouldn't see anyone else. Cass's story was not only unusual for me to hear in such depth, but my guess is that it is for anyone reading too.

I already knew that Lucy was concerned about Cass and that she had felt confused and shut out by his obvious dip in mood. She knew that he hadn't just observed the two miscarriages they had been through and that he was bottling up some difficult feelings. He had been beside her for the first one at home, and again, with her at the scan that revealed their next baby had died. But as he began to obviously struggle, a few weeks after her surgery that he had hated for Lucy to have, she no longer felt him by her side. I made sure that Cass didn't feel pressured to meet with me before agreeing to a session time, but his ambivalence when we first spoke was clear: "I'm okay, really. Lucy's worrying too much, but maybe one session will be useful."

Cass and Lucy had a living child, Freddie, and Lucy had told me that they had done as best as they could to parent as equally as their jobs would allow. Cass had been very involved with Lucy's first pregnancy—attending prenatal classes and reading parenting books—and he had been of main support to her during Freddie's birth, even cutting his umbilical cord. He had later taken unpaid leave to supplement his paternity allowance and spent as much time with Freddie in his early months as he could. He shared Lucy's yearning and planning for another child.

Being a father was, as Cass later described to me, the most

important thing in his life. Even as a little boy, he dreamed of the children he would have and the father he would be. I take these reflections from men for granted now, but it has taken us as a society a long while to realize that fatherhood was in any way psychologically important—both for men themselves and also for their children.

WHILE WOMEN have long been expected to desire motherhood and to become mothers in order to fulfill their ultimate feminine role, men have also been pressured by a cultural pronatalism. The expectation to become a father was more traditionally defined in terms of being a responsible breadwinner for the family—as well as the disciplinarian—rather than adopting the more nurturing, feminine aspects of parenthood: the feeding, soothing, wiping, cooking, and dropping off and picking up from school. These expectations slowly began to change in the second half of the twentieth century, and by the 1980s, a notion of involved fathering had emerged, encouraged by a growing understanding of the psychological importance of fatherhood, increasing numbers of women in the workplace, and a retraction of hospital and extended family care after birth.

My father experienced this shift in expectations in his own lifetime: when my older sister was being born in 1967, he was sent to wait in a room far from the labor ward. My mother would later hold her up against the hospital window so he could see her from the street below—his visiting hours during her then prescribed weeklong recovery were tightly restricted. When my younger sister was born in 1988, he was by my mother's side. I still remember his awestruck face after the event, and he seemed to enjoy his revised skills of diaper changing and bottle feeding. Around the same time, as a seventeen-year-old, I was transfixed by the hugely popular *Man and Baby* poster adorning many of my friends' bedroom walls. Sold by Athena Posters, it showed a shirtless, muscled male model tenderly gazing at the baby he held. I wasn't alone in my fascination at this meeting of masculinity and a typically maternal demeanor—the image sold more than 5 million copies.

In the UK now, 98 percent of fathers who live with the birth mother attend the birth of their baby, and the number of men who act as their children's primary carer has risen tenfold in the last decade to over 700,000. Not a huge number admittedly, but it's still a significant leap. In the US, the number of fathers who are at home with their children has nearly doubled since 1989, to around 2 million. While only 21 percent of these men say the main reason they are at home is to care for their family (as opposed to being unable to find employment or because of illness or disability), this is a fourfold increase from 1989, when only 5 percent of fathers stated the same.

Yet we are in a state of confusion. On the one hand there seems to be an increasing acceptance of involved fatherhood as an ideal, but simultaneously our culture—and its institutions—has been slow to shed some deep-seated ideas about gendered parenting roles. If men do take up the traditionally female child-care role, they can feel a curiosity, or—in the words of a friend of mine—"heroic" for doing so. Some studies suggest that they can feel persistently judged by society as a secondary parent or support partner to the mother of their child, however involved they may be. One area where this tension plays out in the UK concerns how parental leave entitlements are taken up by men, and a committee of MPs recently called for reform after research showed that many fathers feel that their workplace isn't supportive of them taking time away from work to care for their children, even though they are entitled to it.

I DETECTED THAT Cass was caught up in his own version of this unsettled state. While as involved as he could be as a father and father-to-be, he felt he couldn't claim full rights to the potential parenthood that he had lost, and he felt that his distress didn't count as much as Lucy's. This partly explained why he needed encouragement from Lucy to see me, and why he conveyed ambivalence when we first spoke, but men are also far less likely to seek professional help than women when it comes to their health generally, and even more so with their mental health. Men can underestimate how emotionally vulnerable they are actually feeling, and believe that they should both control and guard against this. In recent years, campaign work has picked up on this potentially damaging trend: in the UK, men grow mustaches in November for the annual Movember event to raise awareness of men's health issues and to normalize seeking help for them—including prostate and testicular cancer, mental health issues, and suicide. In early 2018, Prince Harry ignited debates about a male culture of stoicism when he spoke openly about his grief and suffering in the wake of his mother's death.

The national director of Cruse—the UK's leading bereavement charity—agrees that men are reluctant to seek support: only one in every four people who contact the charity are men, and they largely seek information, rather than take up the charity's offer of one-to-one support. If they do seek emotional backup, it is more likely to be via email or phone, or at a support group where they know that other men will be present. In the case of miscarriage, the same seems to apply: men are only occasional visitors to the face-to-face support groups of the Miscarriage Association in London, and they always attend in tandem with their partner. But none of this means that men don't *want* support, but maybe it is in ways that don't suit women.

Cass began our meeting by telling me why Lucy wanted him to see me—a typical start to a meeting with a man about their experience of miscarriage. She was worried that he wasn't sleeping well and that he was losing his temper far more than normal and seemed to be very stressed. Lucy had felt him physically and emotionally withdraw from her and their son, Freddie, and work and his training for a half marathon meant he was away from home even more than usual. It was unlike the couple to be isolated from each other, and rare for there to be no affection between them, and their sex life had ground to a halt.

I coaxed Cass to tell me in his own words how the trial

of recent months had affected him. He took some time to speak freely. "I wish I hadn't been so naive. Everything was plain sailing for us when we had Freddie, so it didn't occur to me that anything could go wrong the second time round. I guessed that Lucy was pregnant before her period was late—she looked different to me. I bought the pregnancy test on the way home from work, and I was the one who saw the result emerge first. We were soon talking about our next baby's future: if it's a girl, would we ban pink clothes? How would Freddie be with a sibling? What would we do differently?"

HEARING CASS TALK THROUGH some of his plans and dreams and hypotheticals powerfully conveyed to me the strength of his bond with his child-to-be—their baby lived vividly in his imaginings, despite his lack of physical connection with the pregnancy. Unlike the relatively new and morphing idea of involved fathering, this paternal bond to a child in mind is far from contemporary. Movingly, the most famous English diarist, Samuel Pepys, began his legendary work on New Year's Day of 1660 by writing about his sadness that he and his wife were not expecting a baby: his wife had not had "her terms" for some seven weeks, but any hope of a pregnancy had been dashed on New Year's Eve, "when she hath them again." There's no way of knowing whether Pepys and his wife suffered an early miscarriage or her period was unusually late, but his disappointment in losing the promise of a child—and he never did have one—was clearly significant enough for him to record it.

Four hundred and fifty years after Pepys, another man of undoubted future historical note, Mark Zuckerberg, the founder of Facebook, wrote about his painful loss of his potential three children. Announcing his wife's pregnancy on his Facebook page in 2015, he also described the devastation of their three previous miscarriages. Unlike Pepys, who wrote in code to keep his thoughts and observations private, Zuckerberg wanted his feelings to be known by the world: "You feel so hopeful when you learn you're going to have a child. You start imagining who they'll become and dreaming of hopes for their future. You start making plans, and then they're gone. It's a lonely experience."

Given it took so woefully long for both researchers and healthcare professionals to realize that women can form strong bonds with their unborn, it's no surprise that it took even longer for their male partner's perspective to be considered. Hugh Jolly, a famous English pediatrician in the mid-1970s, was an influential campaigner (along with Stanford Bourne and Emanuel Lewis) for the better support and care of women after their babies died at birth, but he also made a valuable and relatively unusual point about referring to the grief of husbands, parents, and families in his writings.

In one paper, Jolly described his concern at the "appalling" treatment of families in hospitals after the death of a stillborn baby—referring to babies being taken away after birth, denied any acts of parentage, and disposed of without permission or dignity. Although his impassioned paper concerned cases of stillbirth (which, at that time, referred to babies born dead after twenty-eight weeks' gestation), he didn't forget the experience of miscarriage, concluding: "it is clear that the need to mourn is not necessarily reduced by the fact that the baby has died earlier." Jolly emphasized his concern for the children of bereaved parents, knowing that they may well suffer for their own loss of a potential sibling, but also because the grief of their mourning parents could well have an effect on their parenting too.

In the mid-1980s, a decade after Jolly's impassioned paper, studies began to explore not only the bond between a pregnant woman and her unborn but also paternal-fetal bonding. They are inconsistent in their approach and findings, but some results indicate that men can bond with their baby in the womb in the same way as their partner can. At the very least, this strand of research accepts that pregnancy is often a rich time of psychological and emotional preparation and adjustment for a father-to-be, and it was obvious from the way Cass talked about Lucy's pregnancies that this had been the case from at least the moment he saw the result of each of her pregnancy tests.

Cass was able to participate in the earliest revelation of his much-wanted babies by buying, and then nervously watching, the pregnancy test kits for Lucy—this simple technology has helped many men forge a link to their newly conceived for years now. More recently, smartphone apps have been created to more consciously bring prospective fathers into the mysterious world of their partner's womb. But they strike me as sending mixed messages about a man's place in his partner's pregnancy: while on the one hand they welcome him in, they simultaneously keep him at a comfortable distance. An overwhelmingly gender-stereotyped banter offers snippets of information geared to keep their expectant partner placated or soothed.

One example of these—the Who's Your Daddy app—offers "9 months peace of mind for the price of a small beer," with a timeline for an expectant dad's calendar (such as "research prams this week") and daily tips (at 136 days to go, "Keep telling your partner how beautiful she is"). Meanwhile, the baby's growth is conveyed in terms that men can apparently handle: from the size of a unicorn (and the weight of expectation) at conception to that of a back-scratcher near term. Other comparisons are made with a fishing lure, a Yoda *Star Wars* figure, a hammer, and a beer bottle. While many men may welcome any help across the bridge to their partner's pregnant world—these apps are selling fast—such blokey messages leave little space for the more intimate type of connection that men like Cass may want to feel. Nor do they mention the prospect of, or deal with, pregnancies that truncate by miscarriage.

Although Cass would never be yoked to Lucy's second pregnancy in the literal and visceral way that she was, he spoke of how Lucy's descriptions of her symptoms—and her obvious physical changes—reminded him of his growing baby, just as they did for her. "I felt so awful for Lucy in the early weeks—she was so unwell and exhausted but was still going to work and looking after Freddie as usual. There was so little I could do to make her feel better, apart from help more and feed her strange foods." He couldn't see the physical reality of his tiny baby on a scan or feel its body from the outside, but the ideas of it in his mind lived vividly without effort on his part.

Cass had made every effort to empathize with Lucy's bodily symptoms, so his guilt was fueled when, in the ninth week of her pregnancy, he dismissed her fears that their baby was under threat. "I wish I had taken Lucy more seriously when she woke up that morning feeling something was up. I was trying so hard to be upbeat for her, I even tried to dissuade her from calling the hospital, as there weren't obvious symptoms. But now I keep thinking that if I had taken her to hospital then, before everything started to go so wrong, things could have been different." Lucy was temporarily soothed by a telephone call with a midwife, and she and Cass carried on their day as best as they could. But however optimistic he'd tried to be, Cass remained distracted by privately held fears for Lucy and their baby.

As Lucy was putting Freddie to bed that night, the bleeding they both had been dreading began. Cass described how deep he had to dig to be strong, and to quickly rally help: "I'll never forget the fear on Lucy's face when she showed me her bloodstain. I was so scared too, but I didn't want her to see that, and I knew that I had to sort everything out. When I called Lucy's sister to come over, and then the cab to take us to the hospital, my hands were shaking so much, I could barely do it."

Cass continued to push his terror away as he and Lucy had a long wait in accident and emergency. "We had to sit in a tiny curtained-off cubicle, with so much else going on around us that seemed to be more important. I didn't have a seat to sit on, so I sat with Lucy on the bed, making stupid jokes, trying to distract her. I couldn't believe how long we had to wait—it seemed so cruel when we thought our baby was dying, and Lucy was so frightened. I kept telling her I was looking for a chair, but I was frantically nagging the nurses to hurry the doctor along."

Cass's role as a "supporter and protector"—of both Lucy and their unborn child—often plays out during and after a miscarriage. It may be logistically necessary too: women can be incapacitated by the pain and bleeding that miscarriages frequently involve, and may need someone else to help them out. The stark reality is that hospitals don't always have the resources available for swift and appropriate care, especially in accident and emergency—the lack of a chair for Cass, and his and Lucy's long wait to be attended to, is, unfortunately, not the worst story I have heard or recounted in this book.

One fascinating study of miscarriage in early modern England paints a scene of similarly anxious husbands, doing their best to supplement the care of their wives by the then all-female network of family, midwives, and experienced neighbors. We don't have the evidence to understand in depth how these husbands felt about their unborn—and whether they were driven to protect him or her too—but the authors quote letters showing how husbands sought medical care from others or even medical knowledge for themselves—perhaps the nearest equivalent to taking their wives to accident and emergency.

Extant notes from apothecaries (an early medical practitioner who prepared drugs) record requests from husbands worrying about their wives' reproductive ailments, including copious blood loss after "untimely births," which must have been terrifying for any father-to-be to hear of—or maybe even witness. These husbands, as more likely to be literate, would also be the ones to break bad news. In a moving letter to his mother-in-law in 1631, Sir William Masham, an English aristocrat and politician, tells her that her future grandchild, clearly long awaited, had died: ". . . to let you know of some ill of my wife, who was yonge with child and hath mis carryed this daye. It is the greatest griefe to us, having bene thus long without; I praye God sanctefye this affliction to us."

David supported and protected me while my body let go of our pregnancies; like Cass he called cabs, sorted childcare, and ensured my safe arrival at the various hospitals I attended over the years. There were many times he had to step up when staff levels depleted—he helped me to the loo when bleeding flooded me, caught my vomit in cardboard dishes, and informed nurses of drips running dry. He was the one to break bad news to friends and family and to receive commiserations that were largely directed toward me. These were undoubtedly difficult moments for him, and very few people ask me or him about those times either, but I had the opportunity to ask Cass about them for him.

Cass described how there was little consideration that Lucy was a scared and grieving mother-to-be on the accident and emergency bed, but even less that he was a scared and grieving father-to-be. "Eventually the doctor arrived, examined Lucy, and confirmed our worst fears. I tried so hard not to cry—I had wanted our baby so much. She did talk to Lucy kindly, but she barely looked at me until she sent us home and she handed me an appointment sheet and Tylenol. It would have been good if she had said she was sorry to Lucy, but also if she had said it to me too."

Cass felt helpless in these frantic hours: during their long wait at hospital and later on, back at home. Nothing could soothe his frustration at not being able to ease Lucy's physical pain or stop the inescapable tragedy from happening or, indeed, his own rising grief for the loss of the family they had both been planning for. "I wish we were told about how much it would hurt. There was nothing I could do for her apart from rub her back and hand her water. It was so awful watching her pacing our bedroom, like a caged animal. I didn't know what to do—and there was no happy ending in sight—nothing I could encourage Lucy with."

Cass's sense of powerlessness fed his guilt. He blamed himself for not taking Lucy seriously enough when she first felt things were awry, and for not taking the opportunity to see his tiny baby when Lucy did. "When Lucy knew the baby was coming, I helped her to the bathroom and held her hands as she sat on the loo. But I was too frightened to look at what she scooped up from the water. Lucy feels so guilty for flushing our baby away, but I didn't stop her, and I wish I had. We had nothing to bury, and I regret that now."

I knew that Lucy also felt intense feelings of guilt and self-blame, and the couple shared a similar mixture of sadness, yearning, anxiety, envy, and anger, but Cass felt these at different times to Lucy, and expressed them in different ways. He spoke of his bitterness toward a colleague who excitedly showed him photos of his newly born baby, a day after he had returned to work. He hated pushing Freddie's stroller as he had earmarked it for a replacement. And for weeks, he avoided using the loo that had carried his baby away.

What little research there is on the male response to miscarriage suggests that Cass is not unusual: men can, and do, feel very similarly to their partners, although they tend to show their feelings in different ways and can be hit by some emotions at a later stage than their partner, after "holding it together" for them in the immediate aftermath. Bereavement literature has labeled these different ways of grieving in loosely binary ways, with the typically male "instrumental style" pitted against the typically female "intuitive style." Gender only influences rather than determines these mourning behaviors though, and I'm sure we all know of exceptions to the prescribed camps or of someone who could be described as both, as I could be.

A typically female intuitive griever finds ways to vent her feelings more openly—through crying or talking—and is more likely to seek support from friends and family, or from strangers through support groups, or from professionals such as talking therapists. This certainly applied to Lucy: she had reached out to me and cried in our sessions and with her mother, her sister, and the few friends who got it. Although, on many occasions, she felt a lack of true understanding of her loss—and therefore grief—by others, she at least had an accepted cultural script for the *manner* of her grieving: big girls can cry, even if big boys can't.

Some argue that displays of grief have long been the preserve of women. The author and academic Gail Holst-Warhaft concludes that in parts of ancient Greece, women's defined ritual, and public, mourning role—unleashed and conveyed by their sung laments—became a problem for the city-state. She argues that the strength of the grief and anger for death could end up dissuading men from joining the army, with its noble goal of dying for one's state. Ultimately, it could be unsettling to peace. In Ireland and Scotland, "keening"—haunting, wailing songs of grief—was performed only by women, fading out in the 1950s (although they can be still found on recordings). More recognizably for me, the academic bereavement literature that first emerged in the 1960s and 1970s was largely grounded in studies of women's experiences of losing a husband. Female grief is probably the version we recognize the most—and sometimes, with the judgment for becoming "hysteric" too.

We don't tend to recognize a typically male instrumental griever, like Cass, though—partly because he may well find private times and private places to let his feelings out, but also because male grief has been, traditionally, less well represented in academic and other literature. One bereavement support worker in a busy London hospital told me of her repeated experience of witnessing men cry the moment they stepped out of the hospital room where their baby had died—away from their partner and most staff. Instrumental grievers tend to "do things" in order to cope with their feelings, rather than crying or talking them through. Cass spoke to me of his need to be "useful": "A few days after our first miscarriage, I signed up to run a half marathon to raise money for a pregnancy loss charity. I found comfort in the training schedule, as it gave me a structure when things felt chaotic. And when I couldn't sleep, I'd read all about miscarriage in a desperate—futile—attempt to help us make sense of things."

Dr. Robin Hadley, an academic who researches the male reproductive experience, is convinced, as I am, that our social conditioning plays a significant role in this instrumental grieving style that men often display. He told me that "Women are socially conditioned to be more emotionally expressive and articulate than men. In turn, this helps them to find their ready-made outlets of support more easily or, indeed, find new ones. Our notion of masculinity, however, is very limiting. Although things are beginning to change, many men are brought up to contain feelings—they may be told or encouraged not to cry, or to resolve vulnerable feelings through 'actions.' Ultimately, they can learn to cut off from their emotional world and to rely on their *thinking* in times of vulnerability instead." We both observed a male phenomenon in our consulting rooms: "Ask a man what he feels, he'll often answer 'I think . . .'"

The psychologist Cordelia Fine's popular book *Delusions of Gender* supports this view about social conditioning. She revisited the research and ideas on gendered behaviors to conclude that they are more of a response to our social, cultural, and personal context than anything else. Once we are recognized as male or female, we are then molded in traditionally gendered ways. I saw this happen time and again when I'd point out that my long-haired infant son was not, in fact, a girl: people would distance their bodies, lower their voices a little, and—one time, memorably—someone began to switch the subject to talk about his "inevitable" future love of football.

Foz Foster is a British artist who strikes me as both an instrumental and an intuitive griever. Like Cass, he ran marathons—for the Miscarriage Association—but his grief also played out creatively and more openly. He depicted his experience of his wife's three miscarriages—along with other men's stories he'd researched—in a 75.5-foot scroll painting, *Pain Will Not Have the Last Word*, that wrapped around the walls of the Camden Image Gallery in 2015, not far from where I live in London. The vividly colorful, sometimes childlike painting conveys lost moments Foster had hoped to share with his three potential children, shattering any idea that men don't suffer too. It displays space hoppers and cuddly toys, Mickey Mouse, and the words "Look DAD," as well as three dark pink baby-like figures beneath the moving words "My babies are dead . . . Why did you leave me without saying good bye."

I heard Foz speak about this painting at a public event about infertility, pregnancy loss, and childlessness: his work is political, and he uses it as a platform to tell men's stories all over the country. He talked about his lack of preparation for his wife's first miscarriage, which contributed to his intense shock and helplessness during what he described as such a brutal, visceral experience. He spoke of the well-meaning inquiries from friends about his wife, but never about him: "It seems that it takes two people to make a baby, but only one to have a miscarriage." Hearing him describe his creative process with the scroll left me in no doubt about the depth of relationship he had forged with his lost babies: "It allowed me to play with my miscarried kids. I took them to the fair, played in the park, gave them presents at Christmas." He later told me how the work is also a living memorial for his and other lost children.

SPEAKING WITH Dr. Hadley and Foz Foster brought home to me another social reality that contributes to observed instrumental grieving after a miscarriage: there are few narratives for men to draw on when they talk about their more tricky reproductive experiences in general. While we have a way to go before a parity of parenthood roles fully emerges, we also have some way to go before we fully appreciate the entire emotional realm of the male reproductive experience: all that happens before conception, during a pregnancy, after a birth, and when a miscarriage happens.

The templates that we do have for male reproductive narratives tend to view men as virile from puberty to death (even though factors in the male partner account for about half of the known cases of infertility), as generally subsidiary to the efforts involved in making a baby, and as less emotionally vulnerable than women when they experience infertility and pregnancy loss. I rarely hear about men being broody, when I know they are. Dr. Hadley adds, "It's interesting that in the UK we have a medical college devoted to obstetrics and gynecology but no equivalent one of andrology for a man. Nor do we know how many childless men there are, as only a mother's fertility history is officially recorded."

Without easy ways for men to express their feelings about desiring—and losing—potential fatherhood, this may corrupt how men talk to other men who have not been through similar experiences of loss. One British research paper suggested the same, with a participant quoted as saying, "My mates would only laugh if I broached the subject with them . . . so it's best not to." This was written twenty years ago, and I'm not sure if a response like this would be wholly predictable today, but men can, and do, still hold back from their friends and family for fear of being misunderstood, and some prefer the safer support of fellow male bereaved online.

Those who are willing and able to speak up—like Foster and Zuckerberg—are valuable forces of change: a man giving permission to other men to be vulnerable has a more powerful effect than a woman giving the same. Zuckerberg's candid Facebook post prompted an outpouring of stories of pregnancy loss online and in the print and TV media—as well as 1.7 million "likes" at the time of writing. Not only did his and his wife's story help to raise awareness of miscarriage generally but also his male voice counted for a lot too.

CASS FOUND VERY FEW OUTLETS to talk about his feelings. Just as he felt he couldn't talk about his broodiness before his babies had been conceived, he also felt he couldn't talk about his reluctance to try and conceive again after their first miscarriage. He feared another heartache and the heavy weight of disappointment if they didn't conceive soon or at all. But he didn't want to let Lucy down by getting in the way of her desperate desire to be pregnant once more.

When Cass found out Lucy was—they were—pregnant again, he did his best to balance his hopes and fears, along with supporting Lucy through her own vacillation of feelings. "Waiting for the test felt so differently from before. We had lost our blissful innocence, or ignorance, by then, and I no longer believed that pregnancy meant the inevitability of having a child."

Like Lucy, Cass felt hesitant about bonding with his baby, although as the pregnancy progressed through the ninth week—the time their second baby had died—toward the reassurance of a twelve-week scan, his confidence of being a father again increased. "I was far more vigilant of Lucy's health and happiness this time round. I was distracted at work and just wanted to be near her as much as possible, just in case things went wrong again. There were times I felt sick too, and we joked together if I was having my own pregnancy symptoms in sympathy."

I suspect Cass's nausea was a symptom of stress and anxiety rather than anything else, but rarely, some men do experience their own physical and psychological pregnancy-like symptoms. The English anthropologist Edward Burnett Tylor is the first to have spotted a physiological male response to pregnancy and birth, coining the term "couvade" in 1865, from the French word "*couver*" (to brood or hatch). He observed a number of remarkable behaviors among some of the expectant fathers he lived with in South America and the West Indies, such as withdrawing from their work and social life, and shouting out, as if in pain, during the birth of their baby. They may even have taken their newborn to bed after birth. Tylor concluded that there was a closer physical bond between a father and his baby among these cultures than had been observed elsewhere.

Along with male infertility and the male experience of pregnancy and its losses, the modern phenomenon of "couvade syndrome," or "sympathetic pregnancy," has piqued little sustained interest in the medical and research field. We don't know why it happens, to whom it most often happens, or what could be the cause of it. What thin research there is uses varying definitions of the experience, which makes a coherent inquiry difficult: estimates range wildly between low and high incidences, and the suggested causes also vary enormously.

We also know nothing about what happens to these men after a miscarriage, although one puzzling constant seems to be that men experience couvade largely during the first and third trimesters. It has been relegated in the popular mind to an endearing, if not laughable, phenomenon; in one such example, a British tabloid newspaper in 2012 teases a man for being "wimpy" for his suffering, which (reportedly) included morning sickness, exhaustion, headaches, heartburn, hot flushes, and a swollen belly. When I suffered some of those deeply uncomfortable symptoms myself, no one ever called me a wimp.

Cass's nausea and anxiety waned as the safety of the second trimester beckoned, with its scan at the start to reassure the couple that all was well. Ultrasound scans only became an integral part of the pregnancy health-care package in the 1980s. They were originally developed in the 1930s and 1940s for clinical work on the ventricular spaces in the brain and were later used in World War II to help surgeons operate in the dark. They moved into obstetrics in Glaswegian hospitals in the 1950s and 1960s, used when an abnormality in a baby was suspected, but women weren't allowed to see what was going on: these scans were a purely medical event.

Nowadays, scans are more akin to medical *and* social events, where parents—and maybe siblings or grandparents—meet their new family member, with resulting images often forming a part of family records or archive shared with social networks. Expectant parents can also pay privately, and handsomely, for more sophisticated scans. One company offering such services, enticingly named Window to the Womb, has thirty branches throughout the UK and offers "4-D" scans, plus a movie recording for babies after sixteen weeks: "time" being the fourth dimension at play while you view your baby's 3-D movements.

Studies have emphasized the profound impact of ultrasound imagery on a partner's bond with his unborn—and his subsequent grief when his baby then dies. Along with pregnancy tests, websites, and apps, scans have become another way in which technology allows us a glimpse into the otherwise mysterious world of a pregnant womb. So much of our knowledge these days is mediated through what we see; it seems that we need to see things to believe in them more than we ever did before.

One researcher found in her interviews with eighteen British men that "Visual knowledge . . . became their window or gateway into the interior of the woman's body, and *simply because it was visual* appeared to extend the strongest 'evidence' (their terminology) of the baby." But research has also shown that men can feel excluded from the scanning experience, and the inescapable emphasis on the pregnant woman's body can cloud the fact that another parent is deeply concerned, and connected, with what is revealed.

CASS HAD TAKEN A DAY off work to be with Lucy for their scan, not revealing to his colleagues why. "I spent ages thinking about booking a table for lunch at our favorite restaurant, for after the appointment. I wanted to think it would be a day of celebration, but I worried that it would jinx things, and Lucy felt the same. We were both full of hope and full of nerves, but I didn't want Lucy to know about my nerves."

Cass remembered how he braced himself to see his third baby on the screen. "I was holding my breath from the moment the sonographer started to look at the screen. But it took far too long for her to say anything, and then she told us there was no heartbeat. I couldn't say anything at all—I was struck dumb." I will never forget one quote in a research paper written over twenty years ago from a male participant at a similar moment: "When we were told after the ultrasound that the worst had happened it was like someone had just stuck hot pokers in my sides."

For the second time in just a few months, Cass pushed his shock away to console Lucy—he wanted to of course, but he was also left feeling invisible, and to blame. "The sonographer turned the screen off and left the room. It seemed she had forgotten it was my baby too; I don't remember her looking at me. In my darkest moments, I still wonder whether my original unwillingness to try for that baby was somehow transmitted—that on one level, it knew it didn't feel fully welcomed in the world." He then told me how he helped Lucy to get dressed and then held her back when she tried to turn the screen back on.

The sonographer returned to take the couple outside to the waiting room and told them a doctor would talk to them soon. "Again I found myself desperately wanting a doctor to hurry up—Lucy was quietly sobbing in my arms, and we were among strangers in a crowded room. And when she did arrive, she mainly spoke to Lucy about the next steps. I know it was her body at stake, but it was our baby too. I also hated hearing the word 'management' for what would have to come next—it made no sense to me."

Once they had decided to choose surgery to remove their baby from Lucy's body, Cass had to do what many partners do: relay the bad news to family and close friends. "I dreaded making those calls. Telling people made everything so real, and I had to hold it together. Of course people were rightfully concerned about Lucy and the surgery, but only one person asked how I was—and then didn't wait to hear my full answer. Just because I sounded together, it didn't mean that I was."

Cass's manager was understanding and gave him a week's compassionate leave—as with all miscarriages, of whatever gestation, he wasn't entitled to paternity rights or benefits by law. A week's leave could be seen as generous by some or very unfair by others, but Cass was ready to return after that break anyway. "I wanted to get back to work as I had a big project on—it helped me to keep busy, just as my running helped me too." Keeping busy also meant that Cass could protect Lucy from his own upset. "Lucy was in bits, and she had to go through a physical recovery on top of everything else. It didn't feel fair to burden her—I couldn't talk about how frightened I was that her surgery might go wrong, or how angry I felt with the world. And I didn't want to stir up her own upset either."

Like many men I work with, Cass feared he would drown Lucy's already vulnerable state with the addition of his own feelings. Nearly half (46 percent) of 160 partners (mainly male) participating in a survey commissioned by the Miscarriage Association about miscarriage and ectopic pregnancy said they kept their feelings hidden from their once-pregnant partner, for fear of causing her additional distress or saying the wrong thing, and 22 percent held back from talking about any feelings of loss or pain. In my experience this fear of drowning rarely manifests: women appreciate and draw strength from their partners' sharing of experience with them. This survey also found that partners wanted to talk about their feelings nonetheless—so if men feel they can't talk to their partners, it follows that we should support them to find outlets elsewhere.

Campaign work has long addressed the need to increase the availability of emotional support for women after miscarriage in medical and other settings, and more recently this has been extended to include support for partners. If a man is an archetypal instrumental griever, this may mean thinking about ways to talk and express feelings that differ from those for the archetypal female intuitive one. I know that Cass benefitted from (eventually) opening up to me in a consulting room, and he spoke of the healing conversations he had while running with a friend, and with another who helped him look after Freddie when Lucy was recovering in bed. "Doing"—while talking—suited Cass more than Lucy.

While the couple took incongruent paths through their grief, this meant that they unwittingly created an unhelpful feedback loop of communication that I have come to know well through my work. Cass held back from sharing his feelings with Lucy, and from explicitly asking her about how she was getting on, and Lucy could interpret his apparent aloofness as a lack of care or interest. She could feel isolated and resentful, while Cass felt his own loneliness because of their estrangement. Online, women often let off steam about how their male partners seem to lack understanding or sympathy, but as a forum moderator noted to me, other women often quickly respond to suggest that this may be more to do with different ways of handling their grief than anything else.

Lucy and Cass were ultimately able to iron out the creases that arose between them by learning of each other's versions of events and feelings. In short, they were honest when talking to each other about what they had been going through. Lucy came to appreciate that Cass's apparent disinterest sprang more from fears and a broken heart, while Cass realized that Lucy needed him to share his vulnerabilities, despite feeling the weight of her own. Rather than swamping her as he feared, sharing his feelings lightened the load of her own anguish, and the full understanding they were eventually able to give each other was invaluable.

A US study in 2010 found that parental relationships have a higher risk of dissolving after miscarriage or stillbirth, compared with those after a live birth. Had Lucy and Cass not had a stable relationship to start with, or consciously addressed their problems, or sought help (which doesn't have to be through therapy), their miscarriages may have strained it, maybe even beyond repair. The author Ayobami Adebayo explores the stress of reproductive loss beautifully near the beginning of her novel *Stay with Me*—a story of a childless and crumbling marriage in Nigeria, where the pressure on women, and couples, to have children bears down even more heavily than it does in the West. Akin, the husband of Yejide, reflects, "Before I got married, I believed love could do anything. I learned soon enough that it couldn't bear the weight of four years without children. If the burden is too much and stays too long, even love bends, cracks, comes close to breaking and sometimes does break."

IN MY CHAPTER on late miscarriage, featuring Emma and Jen, I note how relatively little we know about the lesbian experience of miscarriage in the research literature, and how heterosexual norms govern most of our institutional and cultural ideas about reproduction. In my experience of working with lesbian partners after miscarriage, many have described their desire and need to be strong and supportive while a miscarriage took hold of their loved one's body, but in addition, they may well have to contend with social biases in a way that heterosexual male partners never will.

While the role of fatherhood has proven changeable and subject to the lack of certainty we have around the notion of masculinity, at least "father" has a well-defined meaning as compared to the "other mother" of a lesbian couple. Her grief may be discounted by society because of her lack of genetic link with her miscarried baby: some women tell me they have been asked "Are you the 'real' mother?" I've spoken to lesbian couples who have felt abandoned by friends and family because of the assumption—spoken or unspoken—that they can look after each other well enough, because women tend to be better at talking through their feelings and at emotional support more generally.

But as my story of Emma and Jen also showed, for lesbian couples, trying to conceive is always complicated—no happy accidents can happen before their miscarriages either. The exhausting, time-consuming, emotionally draining, and often expensive fertility processes involved in achieving a pregnancy can add up to the same heightened experience of loss described by heterosexual couples when they miscarry after fertility treatments.

In the same way we can serve women better by taking the time to find out what a miscarriage means for them, we also can and should do the same for her partner. Even if a miscarriage doesn't unravel in the body of a parent-to-be, this doesn't necessarily mean that the relationship with the baby, and the grief that follows when it is lost, should matter any less. Nor should we assume that an unavoidable and consciously chosen support role is an easy one to pick up and play out. And even if it *looks like* a partner isn't in much distress—because he or she isn't grieving in the more obvious way that women are typically thought to do—it doesn't take much to find out otherwise.

WHILE THE STRENGTH that Lucy and Cass drew from each other was ultimately crucial for both of their journeys through grief, Lucy was also nourished by the support of her mother. Turning to a mother after a lost motherhood is often a natural thing for women to do. I learned from my sessions with Lucy that her mother had her own, difficult, response to the miscarriages. Of course bereaved parents bear the lion's share of distress, but we barely consider that a miscarriage may affect members of the wider family too, and maybe in ways we have never imagined.

Lucy's mother had two sets of painful feelings she had to navigate her way through: those arising from seeing and hearing her daughter in deep and sometimes inconsolable distress, alongside her own personal grief for the loss of her two grandchildren-to-be. And just as Lucy was, she was concerned for Cass and for Freddie; though only two years old, he sensed his parents' upset and distraction and could understand the repeated word "baby" while not actually seeing one around. Another thread of loss emerged too— Lucy's mother had had a miscarriage when Lucy had been a toddler, but she had never discussed it before: as I know so well, miscarriages often give permission for the telling of other miscarriages.

Like many women thirty years ago, Lucy's mother hadn't talked about what had happened with friends or family or shared her feelings of grief with anyone apart from her husband. The pressure her mother felt then to "shut up and put up" was more intense than what she perceived to be the case for women today—and Lucy was left with no conscious inkling of her sibling-to-be. However, witnessing and supporting her daughter's experiences reawakened the memories of this past loss, and Lucy came to learn the story of another family bereavement that, like her own, would never quite find its bearings.

Lucy had never known that, for most of the years while she was growing up, her mother had privately remembered both the date of her miscarriage and the day she had hoped to give birth to a sibling for Lucy. Neither had her younger sister, born a year after this due date. In more recent years, emboldened by pregnancy loss awareness campaigns, Lucy's mother had bought flowers for the kitchen table to mark her lost due date, but only ever told Lucy's father why. Lucy told me how much she appreciated her mother's candor—as she did other women's too—and how this shared grief supported her. She vowed to talk more to her mother about her experience, not wanting the topic to disappear again.

My mother also had miscarriages after I was born, and I have no doubt that mine touched on her memories of her own losses. Her overwhelming feeling after mine was a tangled mixture of pain for me, for David, and for her lost grandchildren. All my miscarriages upset her, but she was most intimately involved with my first pregnancy, not least because it was so fraught from the outset, involving many hospital admissions and fears. Although already a grandmother, she was excited for her first grandchild from me and David, and then intrigued about a twin pregnancy that she had no personal experience of.

As the babies grew inside me, she began to think about her life with two more grandchildren in her family fold. I shared the news of every frequent scan and every new experience of my rapidly expanding body. She collected some tiny clothes—that she later hid—from a neighbor who had had premature triplets, and often marveled at the idea of two babies arriving at the same time. I remember her excitement at trying out a folkloric gender test, using a strand of my hair looped through her wedding ring to divine grandsons or granddaughters by way of its rotation. Like us, she wondered about names and childcare, double strollers and the prospect of little sleep.

When I began writing this book, I asked her to tell me, for the first time in fifteen years, about the birth of Matilda and Florence from her perspective. I knew that David had called her soon after my labor began and that she kept apprised of my unavoidable journey toward the birthing of two deaths by calling the hospital. "I remember hearing that one baby had been born, but you didn't want to push for the other. That was incredibly painful. I couldn't bear thinking about what you were going through. I arrived at the hospital by the time they were both born and I knew I wanted to see them, but I also knew I had to ask your permission. I remember agonizing over whether to call them 'your' babies or 'the' babies—I didn't know which would upset you more. I thought that you may have wanted to anonymize them, so it wouldn't hurt so much, but I'm glad I chose the word 'your' now."

Given my nonengagement with my labor, and my clear desire at the time not to see the tiny bodies of my babies, my mother's vacillation was entirely understandable. But I learned in our conversation that she had no doubt about their status in the family—they were two of "hers" even if they may have seemed, temporarily, not to have been "mine." By stepping in where we couldn't, she created, and held, a memory of their corporeal existence outside of me until such time when David and I were ready to find out more. She keeps this memory for others too: just as I asked her only recently to tell me more, my father, prompted by my research, also asked her questions about that time that he hadn't before.

My mother had a strong desire at the time to give each of the babies a name. "I knew that they didn't have names then—and we all wrongly thought one was a boy, as your last scan had suggested. But my instinct was to give them names, so that they could go to heaven with them—so that's what I did, in my head. They will always be a part of my life." But despite this being true for my mother, no one ever said to her, "I'm sorry for your loss," as no one treated what had happened as deaths in the family.

When my mother told me of her naming our babies before David and I did, I felt a spark of outrage: she had no right to bestow this symbol of identity on either of them. Nor do I believe in a heaven as she does. But my upset evaporated as quickly as it came, as I appreciated that her private act, at a time of tremendous shock and upset, reflected her firm belief in her granddaughters' status in the world and of her own relationship with them, separate from mine. The names that she chose capped her effort to include them in her

bloodline, as did familiar faces: she describes Matilda's resemblance to David, whereas Florence looked more like me.

Naming often happens months before a birth and is often
tied up with family and memories, as the stories in my previous chapters suggest: Claire and Will named their baby
after Will's grandmother soon after the pregnancy was confirmed; Cass and Lucy discussed possible names on the way
to their fateful scan; while Emma and Jen had spent evening
hours playing the name game. Online memorials for miscarried babies often refer to lost "angels," but there are
countless chosen names virtually inscribed too, however
brief a pregnancy turned out to be. Names are a powerful
means of forging an identity and dignity in the world and
can be a way of continuing family tradition. They can become especially important for a bereaved when the identity
of a dead baby is a precarious one—as is the case in miscarriage. For my mother though, this precariousness was more
around their identity in heaven than on earth.

In researching the psychological importance of naming
babies who have died, I stumbled across a moving case study
of a sibling's experience of a late miscarriage, a perspective
that I hadn't seen referred to in any other literature. Just as a
parent's and grandparent's grief after miscarriage may well
involve the lost imaginings of a future child's life, this narrative shows that siblings can feel the ongoing presence of an
absence. It also shows how siblings can—like my mother did
for me—pick up the role of a keeper of a memory that other
family members may have been unable to inhabit.

As told to a researcher over seven decades after it had

occurred, an Australian woman, Nancy, was born a surviving twin—her sister, small enough to "fit in a choco-
late box" was removed from her mother immediately after
her birth. The tiny size of Nancy's sister suggests that she
had died in the womb long before Nancy's birth—we'll
never know when. As was usual for the time, in 1937, not
only was the baby girl buried in an unmarked grave, but
Nancy grew up knowing nothing more than the barely
mentioned fact of her sister's death. She wasn't embedded
in any family narrative but had been—through convention
rather than desire on Nancy's part—written out of it
instead.

Although her sister's memory hadn't been kept alive by
her parents, extended family, or community, it had clearly
never left Nancy's mind or heart. She described times when
she felt her twin's absence more strongly than others—such
as when she traveled across the world to visit extended family in the UK, in her thirties. I'm guessing that she then felt
a strong desire for a lifelong companion to share her adventures with, and to feel protected and understood by.

Researchers, theorists, and clinicians like myself now
know that continuing a bond with a loved one after their
death is both a typical and indeed a healthy part of the grieving process. As was the case with Nancy, we are now also
acknowledging that this bond can exist between siblings
who may not have ever known each other. In Nancy's case,
she arguably did know her sister from their days in the
womb together—but we have yet to know if, and how,
these memories are stored.

Nancy and her two brothers had made fruitless efforts

over the years to trace their sister's burial place, and many decades later, with the help of a family friend, she was, at long last, successful. She described feeling like she had "won the lottery": a remarkable way to sum up how monumental this discovery must have felt. She was helped enormously by the friend's suggestion that she could name her twin sister, and she chose Catherine after her paternal grandmother, just as she had been called Nancy after her maternal grandmother.

Nancy arranged for a headstone to be set, inscribed with Catherine's full name and dates of birth and death, and on what was her—and would have been Catherine's—seventy-third birthday, a priest gave a graveside blessing ceremony. For Nancy, a practicing Anglican, this ritual from a religious minister played an important part in her mourning for Catherine, becoming a form of consolation, as funeral rites often can be. She poignantly stated, "I will be happy now that Catherine's birth is acknowledged."

Another bigger piece of research picks up on this need for siblings to have their "ghost" sibling acknowledged. It involved interviews with forty-nine adults who had experienced the death of a sibling they never knew—most of whom had died before the age of one, but some who had died during pregnancy. When asked if they had any recommendations for families going through similar bereavements, two-thirds suggested that families should be open, have pictures or somehow remember the child who died. Over half described feelings of sadness or grief in relation to the death—including a grief about how life would have been different had their brother or sister survived.

In her popular book about sibling relationships, *My Dearest Enemy, My Dangerous Friend*, the psychologist Dorothy Rowe impresses on us the overlooked impact of a hidden family death—which a miscarriage so often becomes. She notes that just because a child doesn't know he once had a sibling or sibling-to-be, it doesn't mean it won't affect him or her. Furthermore, "How the parents have interpreted that death, whether it was caused by illness or accident, miscarriage or abortion, greatly affects the child. . . . The fact that there was once someone like me but not me is something to puzzle over and take into account."

I know that my two sons occasionally think about their lost siblings, because they ask me about them. They ask about them because I have made a point of including them in our family story. They know that my maternal love is not for them alone, and as they have grown older, they have come to understand that my ongoing anxiety for their safety, and a spoken gratitude for their aliveness, has its tenacious roots in the pregnancies that did not thrive. Because each son was born and survived after other babies didn't, they also muse on the impossibility of knowing if they would even exist had our lives panned out differently: miscarriage can confront us with some mind-boggling, not always comfortable, "what-ifs."

It is clear to me that the ripples of bereavement after miscarriage have the potential to go further than we tend to anticipate, let alone acknowledge. And while they may lose strength over familial distance, they may well be worth considering nonetheless. I have touched on only the experience of a miscarrying woman's partner, mother, and other child, but there are others too: a brother or sister or even good friend. They may well be grieving the loss of a much-wanted baby, alongside their own difficult efforts to support the mother they care for too.

Six

Efforts to Remember, Pressure to Forget

FUNERALS, MEMORIALS, CAMPAIGNS

Choosing to remember is not a neutral choice.
The commitment to remember, especially in the
face of subtle and not-so-subtle pressures to
forget, is clearly understood by bereaved parents
to be an honourable, moral choice.

—Linda Layne, *Motherhood Lost*

There's often little choice in remembering a miscarriage. For the once-pregnant woman, it is an inevitable, and unchosen, mental act: the trauma of their physical experience may replay in their mind for months and even years to come. Women often know the time and day their pregnancy first became threatened, what they were wearing, and what they were doing. They remember the blood, the clots, the pains, words that were said to them, and things that were done to them. But these recollections can be just a part of a much bigger, more complex memory: of the baby they may never have seen or the one they held in their hand or the one they placed in the crook of an arm. This is the baby annotated with yearned-for dreams, hopes, and imaginings of a future life too—a difficult-to-quantify, privately held memory of memories.

But as a culture, we don't make remembering a miscarriage an easy thing to do. As we can deny the existence and profound nature of a treasured relationship with a baby lost to miscarriage—especially if its embodiment had barely begun—we can also respond awkwardly, and dismissively, to keeping its memory alive forevermore—especially if its embodiment had barely begun. Our recognition of and participation in the efforts to remember a child in mind are inextricably bound up with our acknowledgment that a loved one existed at all. As we puzzle over the status of parenthood, babyhood, and whether a birth actually happened after miscarriage, when it comes to remembering, we also puzzle over what it is we bring to mind, and whether a death actually occurred.

Our efforts to remember have another, more uncomfortable dimension to them: none of us like thinking too closely about the handling and disposal of our own dead bodies, but even more so when it comes to those of our miscarried babies. Unless a baby is lost in a late miscarriage, when its body has become recognizably one to mourn, people can find it disconcerting, or even odd, that the bereaved may wish to perform a ceremony for a baby that is barely embodied, and may not even have been kept. Many early miscarriages happen at home and, as my stories have shown, are then flushed away. The journalist Hadley Freeman touched on this cultural unease when she wrote about her miscarriage in 2017 in the *Guardian*. Before her surgical management, a nurse asked her if she wanted "it" to be cremated or "disposed of" by the hospital and that "People are horrified when I tell them this detail."

We don't ask about funeral rituals, ceremonies, or any type of memory-making that happen after miscarriage, nor do we tend to know that they commonly exist, which is why I want to tell you about them—both as a conclusion to my book and also as a reminder of its beginning, where I hope to convey the power of a relationship with a baby that may reside in only dreams or for a short while in a womb. How we choose to mark the loss of our miscarried baby and to commit to honoring its memory speaks of the strength or type of bond we forged with it—and the love we may well have felt too. But of course the two aren't inextricably bound, and not every bereaved feels the need to outwardly express their desire to never forget.

It's not just a cultural awkwardness that has made it difficult for the bereaved to remember—disturbing hospital practices in the past in the UK have denied untold numbers of parents the opportunity to choose what they wanted to do with their miscarried babies. But things have, thankfully, begun to change, and Freeman writes at a time of new hospital practices, led by revised official guidance. At long last, on an institutional level, it is now understood that the bereaved should be given the opportunity to remember as best they can, rather than instructed to forget.

MANY WOMEN I talk to *want* to remember but also, psychologically, *need* to: in fact, often, their greatest fear can be that their baby will be forgotten. Claire, the client whose story I tell in my first chapter, felt this keenly, even though the baby she lost was fleshed out in far more detail in her mind than in her womb. She· suffered her miscarriage at home, in her bathroom, in the ninth week of her first pregnancy, conceived after many months of trying and after the heartache of repeatedly dashed hopes. She and her partner, Will, had named their baby Maggie —she was sure it was a girl, even though she couldn't know for certain.

I met Claire for the first time a couple of months after her loss, and we spent some time talking through the complex and tenacious feelings that took hold in her grief. Her mind had barely stopped reliving the physical pains that had unfurled in her body that day or let go of all the lost yearnings that had filled her dreams for months. But her aching sadness, loneliness, and despair had been a largely private and lonely endeavor, and the idea of creating a ritual to mark her baby daughter's existence was prompted by my gentle suggestion.

We don't usually wait so long to mark the deaths of other loved ones, but as there was no established cultural or religious ritual available to Claire and Will, it's no surprise that it took my suggestion to encourage Claire's thoughts further. Our lives are peppered with rituals that we may not even be aware of. I like one definition for ritual by an existential psychologist, Tatjana Schnell: "a formalised pattern

of action for constructing meaning from a personally relevant event"—maybe it's the same route we walk to work or
a Christmas pudding recipe we follow each year or, as I
know so well, how some clients settle into the room with me
in weekly therapy. Rituals also provide a sense of order and
structure in our ongoing negotiation with the chaos and
plentiful not-knowing in our lives, which applies especially
in the potential free-wheeling despair after a miscarriage or
miscarriages.

We all know of the well-established communal rituals
that mark and make memories of life transitions such as
birth, marriage, and death. We announce births in news-
papers, send flowers and gifts to the hospital, and later celebrate them with a brit, baptism, or naming service—we
may even throw a baby shower before a baby is born. When
a life ends, we announce the death too and arrange cremations, burials, memorials, and wakes or a practice of shivah.
Unlike baby showers, funeral rituals are far from a modern
practice—Neanderthal burial sites from nearly fifty thousand years ago have been discovered with tools, ornamental
shells, and even food left for dead (assumed-to-be) loved
ones. But neither the rituals around pregnancy or birth nor
those around death have yet to develop confidently when
they are at odds in a miscarriage: it fails to complete these
rites of passage, wavering in a perplexing and uncomfortable state.

As a psychotherapist, I know how important death rituals and lasting acts of memorial can be in helping our grief to
be as healthy as it can. They aid us in affirming the bond we
had with our lost loved ones and convey our ongoing desire

to continue this bond through remembering, as well as marking a profound transition between a life "before," and a life "after." But Claire and Will faced what the bereavement literature describes as an "ambiguous loss" that makes doing any of this especially hard, all the more so if you want your friends and family to participate.

An ambiguous loss is defined as a "unique, unclear, traumatic, externally caused type of loss that has relational implications"; one of these four factors alone, or in combination, will always apply to miscarriage. Miscarriages are tethered to their own context; it's rarely known what happened to cause it; it can certainly be traumatic—especially if surgery or tremendous blood loss is involved; and as my stories show, the "relational implications" can be profound and far reaching. Our ambiguous losses also generally refer to a cleave between the physical and psychological realm: Maggie may have been physically absent from Claire's story, but she was psychologically very present. Where there is a physical presence and psychological absence—such as when a loved one suffers from dementia or addiction—many bereaved can feel misunderstood and alone in their grief as well.

When Claire's aunt had died from cancer, a few years previously, the lack of ambiguity around her death meant it was less problematic for Claire to think about what happened next. It was an accepted death in the family, with a clear protocol for the chosen method to dispose of her body, and there was a swift and collective agreement that a ceremony should follow in which friends and family could reflect on and share with each other stories of her life of six decades. But Maggie's death didn't prompt such obvious steps, nor was there a life to talk about in retrospect—just a potential one that only Claire and Will knew intimately, because no one else had thought to be curious about it.

Even if Claire and Will had been religious, they wouldn't have easily found an established death ritual for an unborn. In nearly all religions, there are clear procedures for an adult death, but barely anything is said about the death of a baby, let alone a miscarried one. Strictly speaking, prayers are not usually offered to children under six years in Islam, shivah is not practiced for a Jewish baby who has died before thirty days, and unbaptized babies have historically been deprived entry to heaven by the Catholic Church. Anecdotally, I know that such strict theological rules aren't always followed by rabbis, Catholic priests, and imams, and one recent study notes how American Catholicism has become more responsive toward pregnancy-loss memorialization, with communities drawing on Catholic rituals and symbols in various ways—including bespoke memorial church services. The Miscarriage Association website tells visitors about other online resources that guide ceremonies, including those offering Jewish prayers and rituals, as well as suggestions for Muslim prayers and practice.

Many hospital chaplains support the bereaved after miscarriage—either by leading a memorial service for pregnancy loss at a hospital or at a funeral service, or by offering emotional help. One friend of mine told me of an annual service her local vicar holds for bereaved parents for all babies lost in pregnancy at a tiny village in rural Norfolk. But despite these acts of empathy and help, it seems that some Christians feel an unease with the Church's overbearing emphasis on having a family life, which makes it difficult for those who have suffered reproductive loss or infertility—or who choose not to have children—to be feel fully included.

Saltwater and Honey is a popular online support website and blog platform set up to help Christians—and non-Christians—through the pain of pregnancy loss, infertility, and childlessness. In a moving and passionate "Letter to the Churches" in November 2017, Lizzie Lowrie, who co-founded the resource, sets out how she has learned that Christians all over the world "have fallen away from the church and sometimes from faith because they believe their grief, their singleness and their childlessness doesn't belong in church." On another web page, she offers a detailed "liturgy of loss"—for a vicar, pastor, or priest to lead a service with—or for the bereaved to consider alone.

Although neither Claire nor Will wanted direction from traditional religions, my sense was that Claire benefited, in her thinking at least, from a growing cultural practice of marking life's transitional events more than ever before. The tragedy of Princess Diana's death has become a noted turning point in the traditional British reserve in response to death, with weeks of spontaneous and highly emotional expressions of mourning from the nation. But since then—and as a result of other cultural shifts—it's much more than death that is acknowledged with ceremony in this country: school proms are now the norm in UK high schools, and more than one of my clients has thrown a party to celebrate the finalization of a divorce. A progressive rabbi, Deborah Brin, writes about healing rituals she has performed for domestic violence, rape, and incest—as well as one for pregnancy loss.

Claire puzzled over what she could do for Maggie: "It feels odd to have nothing to hold on to but our dreams. The only things I had to prove she existed were the four pregnancy sticks and my diary that I kept during the few weeks of my pregnancy. I had hoped to give it to her one day as a gift, so she could see how much she was loved." She instinctively knew that she wanted to use these material things in a ceremony, and I encouraged her: so-called "linking objects" can play an important part in a grieving process, especially when connections to a dead baby can feel so tenuous or sparse.

It used to be thought that using these objects or keeping them could complicate mourning, but it's now accepted in bereavement work that such tangible connections can help the bereaved mourn, rather than make them feel worse. We can still get this wrong after miscarriage—well-meaning friends and family can assume it's helpful to remove any trace of a baby-to-be from the home. In Emma and Jen's story, I note the pain unwittingly caused when a friend removed their daughter's baby things from their home before they got home from the hospital. I, however, hid things away because I couldn't cope with their presence.

Claire brought a small homemade cotton bag to one of our sessions. She was tentative, and clearly uneasy with what it portrayed. "I've been carrying this around with me for weeks—as crazy as it sounds, it has been giving me comfort." Inside, there was one of her pregnancy sticks, with faded proof of Maggie's conception, along with a letter she had written to Maggie a few weeks after her miscarriage, which she read to me. She had inscribed the joy at finding out she was pregnant, the excitement of telling her parents about their grandchild-to-be, and how her name came to be chosen. She emphasized how Maggie would always be remembered, however little known she had been.

Claire's instinct to create this keepsake bag out of the few tangibles she had from Maggie's hidden life reflects a growing practice of remembrance that has been taken up by the bereaved in recent years. A number of small charities now prepare and send memory—or keepsake—boxes directly to bereaved parents who have found them online. But they also supply boxes to more and more hospital units that care for women after pregnancy loss in the UK, and at least one early pregnancy unit makes them too. One charity, SiMBA (Simpson's Memory Box Appeal), prepares three-sized boxes for hospitals, and the bereaved directly, saying on their website "We would suggest our large Memory Box for a loss of a baby over 24 weeks gestation, our medium box for a loss between 14–24 weeks gestation and our smallest box for a loss of less than 14 weeks gestation."

The smallest box reflects the fact that memories are hard to create and collect for the majority of early miscarriages, when parents are unlikely to have spent time with their baby. It offers a number of carefully considered objects, including: a small knitted teddy, butterfly, and blanket; two butterfly charms; a wooden star ornament; a "Just to Say" card for a memory to be inscribed on; and a "Birth Acknowledgement Certificate" for the details of a date or name to be noted on. Butterflies appear as a popular motif of commemoration among the pregnancy loss community: beautiful, fragile, and fleeting, they perhaps capture a sense of what was lost.

If the miscarriage was a later one, the bigger medium-sized box reflects the fact that parents may be better able to capture memories of a baby's body and time spent with him or her. This prepared SiMBA box includes a photo folder with a digital memory card; kits to make hand- and foot-prints with clay or by a non-spoiling inkless method; and a baby wash and blankets. Two Touched by You blankets are also provided for the baby and a parent—to be swapped over at the time of a final good-bye. The overall emphasis is on gathering as many memories—and linking objects—as possible during the short time parents have with their baby. One staff member I spoke with described to me how she was able to make footprints of a baby born at thirteen weeks' gestation.

Of course, memory boxes don't suit everyone, and as with each and every phase of a miscarriage experience, hospital staff are, rightly, trained to prize the choice the bereaved make as to whether they want one—and to keep the opportunity open for a change of heart. My miscarriages happened before the practice of offering them was routine for late miscarriage in labor wards, and I think I would have rejected one at the time—as I rejected much else. I spoke of this with a bereaved mother and writer, Clare, who contacted me after she found out about my writing this book on Twitter. She generously spoke with me about her experiences of the time her baby daughter Delilah died, including the commonly shared one of feeling misunderstood, silenced, and even shunned in her grief. She felt deeply ambivalent about the memory box offered to her by a member of the staff in her hospital in Scotland.

For Clare, the small container was reductive of the trauma of her recent experience and was in no way able to match her anguish and memories of nurturing Delilah inside of her. She told me how she was bothered by the materiality of something "to keep or not keep"—and that she would never have chosen the color pink. In her beautiful poem "Gift Wrapped," she conveys some of this: "Fresh and newborn pink / wrinkling my forehead, / pulling her back in with suction ropes of love. / I am my own vessel, I am her holder / making shapes of her without need / of the four sides of this puzzle." Clare told me of the private ritual she performed for Delilah, alone in the wilds near her home, and she continues to remember her through her writing, as others, like you now, may remember her through reading about it.

MY CLIENT CLAIRE'S bespoke memory bag may have signaled an absence of materiality in Maggie's little life, but this in no way reflected a lack of entitlement to a proper ritual of remembrance. Many couples find ways to do the same for their embryos created during IVF—but again, not everyone understands this desire, and need, to remember. I called the UK organization that regulates fertility procedures—the Human Fertilisation and Embryology Authority—to find out more about commemorative practices that I had been told about, such as the burial of extra, unused embryos and candlelit vigils for those who were used but didn't implant in the womb. Speaking with a spokesman from the media department, I referred to a story I had read about a couple in Australia who have pioneered the manufacture of keepsake jewelry, with at least fifty pieces made with extra embryos from IVF cycles since 2014. Sadly, the response I got for this was a laugh. To be fair, he did swiftly apologize, but he'd clearly missed the point.

Apart from Will, I was the only one to witness the carefully curated contents of Claire's keepsake bag or even to participate in a conversation about how the couple could, and would, create a private ceremony. She had mentioned to a couple of close friends that she was thinking of doing so but had sensed their surprise because of the awkward silence that followed. Just as people may struggle to understand the strength of a bond with an unborn baby, it follows that they may pause in the face of an intention to make an occasion out of it. Claire reflected upon these unwelcomed responses, "I knew then that we weren't going to ask anyone else to join us."

Claire found some inspiration among the many ideas shared among pregnancy-loss communities, personal blogs, and pregnancy-loss charities. These suggestions for marking a loss after miscarriage often symbolize the transience of parenthood and babyhood, and all that goes with this lost future. Bubbles and balloons are released and then drift out of view, candles and lanterns are lit then slowly burn out, and the power of nature is often harnessed—butterflies included. A thoughtful friend gave me a flowering plant after my third miscarriage, infused with a hope of transformation and a sense of the changing seasons. Her wisdom at the time was remarkable—she turned up at my house, uninvited, to give it to me, and said: "This is to help remember your baby by. I don't have to stay, but I'd like to hear how you are." I know of many other such special plants, flowers, and even trees, embedded in London gardens.

The online suggestions as to how to commemorate a baby lost to miscarriage have developed in response to a wider cultural deficit. I'm often moved by this kind of exchange of information, siphoned off from funeral homes, chaplain offices, and the generally brief condolence conversations with friends and family. These heartfelt postings convey no ambiguity, precariousness, or uncertainty: they always commit to what has been lost, affirm the significance of what happened, and uphold the memories that underscore both.

Claire was shored up by the ideas she had researched, and three months after her miscarriage, she and Will made a trip to their favorite beach on the Welsh coast. They built a small fire, then burned the letter she had written to Maggie, and as the wind took away the ashes, she felt a "release" of a "death" that few people were certain had happened. Will then gave Claire a gold letter *M* pendant on a necklace. This reminded me of a moment beautifully described by the rabbi Deborah Brin, who writes about a ritual she performed for pregnancy loss as "an elongated moment, a moment squeezed for all it is worth to make a memorable distinction between what came before and what comes after." If anyone later asked Claire what the *M* stood for, she would sometimes answer the truth, sometimes lie, and at other times fudge her answer: it all depended on whether she could rely on being met with understanding and curiosity or their opposites.

MY WORK WITH Claire stopped soon after her beach ritual had committed her and Will to remember Maggie forevermore. Lucy and Cass had a different experience of and opportunity for making and setting memories. Their first miscarriage had happened at home, and, like Claire, Lucy had regretfully flushed her baby away, as she was flooded by terror, shock, and panic. While the couple had no doubt that they wanted to remember their baby, they assumed, as Claire had, that formally marking their loss would be an out-of-place, even weird thing to do. But when Lucy's second miscarriage was "managed" by surgery, her hospital's response to her baby's death suggested that she would be far from weird to want to mark her loss. Unlike their experience with a couple of doctors, and some friends and colleagues, Lucy and Cass were then encouraged by the hospital staff to nurture the memory of their baby, and *not* to forget.

Before Lucy's surgery, a dedicated member of the staff took time to explain what they could do with the baby who would be removed from Lucy's womb. There was no hurry to decide either, as the hospital could look after the baby for them for at least a couple of months. Like Claire did, many bereaved need some time to work out their wishes. Following new guidelines, staff told the couple that the hospital could arrange and pay for a cremation or burial—either of which could be individual or shared with other miscarried babies. What the guidelines also suggest, although it is hardly ever offered, is the option to dispose of a baby by "sensitive" incineration—which, in practical terms, means separately from other clinical waste.

But these new sensitive disposal options are not offered to everyone in the UK: the guidance in place has yet to be uniformly interpreted across hospitals, and preliminary research suggests there is great room for improvement in implementing and communicating these choices to the bereaved. Lucy and Cass were lucky that the resources of the hospital meant that they had a wide choice—it may well be that a shared cremation or burial is the only option. They were also informed—as they should be—that they could take their baby home with them to make their own arrangements with a funeral director or to bury their baby themselves (with guidance as to where). They were also lucky to face their unenviable choice at a radically improving time of hospital practice: we have a shameful past when it comes to the handling and treatment of our miscarried babies' bodies.

HISTORICALLY, hospitals retained power over babies lost in pregnancy, and conveyed their ownership by, in the case of early miscarriages, taking then disposing of them by incineration along with other clinical waste. For late miscarriages, the hospitals could place the bodies in unmarked and untraceable graves, without any discussion with their bereaved patients. On an institutional level, this excruciating practice sent a powerful signal that such babies should be forgotten, and I've explored in my chapter on late loss how this was bound up with the associated belief that mothers—and their husbands—should not see or hold their babies after they were born. "Forgetting" was deemed best for their recovery in grief and for their preparation to have another child.

This practice of treating once-loved bodies in a such a dehumanizing way, without permission, has a deeply uncomfortable precursor in English history too. In eighteenth-century London, when the demands of anatomists and pathologists increased as their professions established and grew, graves of the very poor were commonly robbed for the sake of the pursuit of knowledge. The ensuing public outrage caused by these body snatchers led to the passing of the 1832 Anatomy Act, which aimed to resolve the competing demands of science and social sensibilities by allowing only unclaimed dead bodies—again, generally of the very poor—to be released and cut open for science.

Nearly two centuries later, it was the strength of public outrage that also led to a shake-up in the practices around the handling and disposal of miscarried babies. Our current guidelines emerge from scandals unearthed by journalists and from campaign work by and on behalf of the bereaved, who championed for parents to be given the choice of a dignified good-bye to a baby that was loved and lost—however gestationally young. Commentators trace the inklings of a shift in paradigm—from hospital ownership to parental choice—to the influential Polkinghorne Report of 1989, which set out to revise the thinking about the use of fetuses and "fetal material" for research purposes. Remarkably it notes: "On the basis of its potential to develop into a human being, a fetus is entitled to respect, according it a status broadly comparable to that of a living person."

After this report, the NHS responded with new guidelines for its staff, stating that disposal of fetuses after miscarriage should be both "sensitive" and "respectful"—which meant, in concrete terms, seeking consent for a cremation or burial where possible, rather than incineration with general clinical waste. Practices were slow to change, and the reputation of some hospitals became mired by the body parts scandal in 1999, when it emerged that organs of children had been removed from their bodies without the consent or knowledge of their parents. Further revelations emerged of the retention and storage of babies lost to miscarriage or stillbirth.

This national disgrace—and its investigations and resulting reports—ultimately led to the passing of the 2004 Human Tissue Act: a legislative framework for issues relating to whole body donation and the taking, storage, and use of human organs and tissue, including all that is lost from a womb in a miscarriage. Pregnancy remains (including fetal tissue) of less than twenty-four weeks are, legally, deemed to be part of a woman. Despite supporting guidance for sensitive disposal of miscarried babies that was published around the time of the act, journalistic endeavors ten years down the line, in 2014, exposed hospitals that were routinely ignoring it and burning fetal remains by their incineration processes without consent of their patients, along with other clinical waste. In some cases, the incinerations had helped to generate hospital power, a fact so shocking that I couldn't engage with the news at the time.

The resulting media storm and public outrage was ultimately fruitful—and Lucy and Cass were just two of the beneficiaries. Hospitals now have four sets of guidance documents (from the Human Tissue Authority, Royal College of Nursing, Institute of Cemetery and Crematorium Management, and Sands charity) that make it clear that remembering—or forgetting—a baby lost to miscarriage is no longer up to them but should be a choice for the bereaved to make and one for hospital staff to communicate clearly about and discern with sensitivity and respect.

As Lucy and Cass were, the bereaved should now be informed of the options available at the hospital for the disposal of their miscarried baby, and depending on the resources available (that do vary from hospital to hospital), this can be by cremation or burial (either individually or jointly with other babies) at the arrangement and expense of the hospital or by sensitive incineration—which means separated from clinical waste. And as mentioned above, women and couples should also be informed that their babies can also be taken home for private arrangements.

Sensitive incineration is an option that many staff find uncomfortable to talk about and very few hospitals actually offer; the Institute of Cemetery and Crematorium Management considers it "unacceptable," and the practice is similarly described in guidance to the Scottish NHS (where abhorrent practices were discovered by the press). If a patient chooses not to decide what to do with their miscarried baby or "pregnancy remains," this probably means that they will be cremated or buried nonetheless—maybe even, in one case I know of, with the blessing of a hospital chaplain. This is a sea change from previous practice and arguably a new sort of paternalism.

My missed miscarriage in 2008 happened before hospital staff routinely addressed disposal options, as they are supposed to now. After waiting a week for my body to let go of my dead baby, there were still no signs of it doing so, and surgery became my only option. Then it was routinely called an evacuation of retained products of conception. I remember signing a consent form for the procedure, but no one asked us to consider what I wanted to do with the "products of conception" once they had been "evacuated": they weren't worth remembering then. Looking back, this was especially odd given I had been handed both of my tonsils when they were removed when I was seventeen and, many years later, my gnarled fallopian tube too.

The surgical management of this miscarriage was a universe away from the birth of my twins six years before—even though it was a few floors above the same labor ward. A midwife had put some pressure on David and me to see our twins, and then offered to arrange a cremation for us, which we hurriedly agreed to. Six years later, I was far from encouraged to remember another, much tinier baby, removed rapidly in a procedure done by rote—and David wasn't considered at all. What I remember most from that deeply unpleasant day was the unflinching stony face of the anesthetist, as my sobs got in the way of his work.

It was heartening to learn that Lucy and Cass's experience was so different from mine and that of untold numbers of other women and partners. They had been spoken to with compassion, they had choice, and they had time to consider how best to cap their memory of their miscarriage experience. But this is not universal. I still hear stories of staff missing the appropriate mark of sensitivity around disposal: for example, a couple who took their miscarried baby into accident and emergency only to be barked at by a nurse, "What do you want us to do with it?" Another woman was told—with little apology—that her baby had been "mislaid" after its surgical removal.

LUCY AND CASS left the hospital after Lucy's surgery with time to take stock of their feelings and to talk further together about what to do. They agreed that they wanted an individual cremation, rather than one shared with other babies lost in the same hospital—an option that was also offered to them and could, in some hospitals, be the only option. This would be at the cost of the hospital, which was also a relief. They had factored in saving money for a new stroller but they hadn't budgeted for a funeral, and while there are many funeral directors who don't charge parents for the funeral of a child or infant or miscarried baby, there are others that do.

The couple wanted to attend a funeral service for their baby alone, but other parents like the idea of babies being together in death and so choose a communal rite—also reflected movingly in "baby garden" sections of cemeteries. One academic in the field of death and bereavement, Kate Woodthorpe, has written a moving paper about the management of these gardens by cemetery and crematoria staff—a unique contribution to a field that is lacking in research. She has found that while we often use "lying down" or "sleeping" to describe interred adults, a different metaphor was used by parents for interred babies that drew on their desire for them to have a playful community together—just as they would if they were alive in nurseries, playgrounds, and schools. This is manifested in toys and other colorful artifacts decorating gravestones (and causing some issues for cemetery staff).

Unlike David's and my experience, Lucy and Cass were told of the place and time of the cremation, so that they could attend the service. Parents don't always want to attend, may not be able to attend if a cremation or burial is a shared one, or simply may not be told—errors in communication can, and do, happen. They had previously discussed with the hospital what to inscribe on the plaque of the tiny coffin, about a foot long, and arrived at the crematoria to see its tiny form already placed on the catafalque—a platform specially made to support a coffin or casket during a funeral service.

Lucy read a poem out loud to those in attendance—Cass, her parents, her sister, and a hospital chaplain. They had felt awkward asking friends and family to attend: funerals for miscarried babies aren't ones that we tend to know about, let alone take time off work for. There was no eulogy to prepare about a life with good innings, nor could the couple share memories of a life spent on earth. The chaplain then performed an act of committal and the couple said their good-bye and set their intention never to forget. Lucy told me they now keep the ashes at home, in a little red urn. Hadley Freeman also tells us about the ashes of her baby—after retrieving them, in a bag, from a crematorium in staggering terms: ". . . I picked up the bag—full of birth and death, love and fire, all the stuff of life—and went home."

My conversations with clients about funerals for their miscarried babies are relatively recent ones: this part of the miscarriage story was long not on the agenda of care. I wanted to learn more about them, not least because of my ignorance about the cremation for our twins, which we weren't invited to. I spoke with three funeral directors and a superintendent at a crematorium about this sensitive work. Words can easily become euphemisms, or even disappear, when we speak of miscarriage, but it was interesting to hear my interviewees' language. They uncomfortably referred to legal and technical terms—"fetus" or "nonviable fetus," "fetal or pregnancy remains"—and relied with far greater ease on the word "baby" or "child."

It became clear that a woman's "bodily tissues"—as our legislative framework describes miscarried babies—becomes a loved and lost person once it arrives at a funeral home. The most recent guidance for burial and cremation authorities, published in 2015, may partly explain what I was hearing. It states its position in stronger terms than hospital guidance—which makes sense given a decision to remember, with a funeral, has already been made by this stage. Early on, it notes "From the parents' point of view, a miscarriage is as significant and devastating as a stillbirth. The baby they were expecting has died and their grief can be profound and long lasting therefore when speaking to parents the term 'baby' must be the only term used." Funeral directors also know what I know when they meet the bereaved: the power of love for the baby who has died in their world, if not in the world outside of the funeral home.

Crematoria now keep a register of miscarried babies they have handled: no one wants a repeat of the past, when many miscarried babies, with no paper trail, were lost without trace. A baby's body is transported to a funeral home from a hospital with a designated member of its bereavement team, a chaplain, or a funeral director. This may be by private ambulance or even a hearse: it doesn't matter that the coffin barely fills it or that a baby may not have a name. But it does matter, a lot, that a baby arrives in a dignified state—both in a suitable container and wearing clothes.

LeighAnne Wright is a funeral director who also runs a charity, Little Things & Co, that, at the time of writing, supplies (for free) more than thirty-one hospitals with clothing for babies born too small for shop-bought clothes. She told me how a bereaved parent sparked her charitable work: "A few years ago, especially before the new guidelines, there was no dignity at all. I would receive babies wrapped in tissue paper or even lying in hospital kidney dishes. One mother just couldn't get past the fact that her twenty-week-old baby had arrived at my funeral home naked. I suggested making a garment for her baby to wear at his cremation, which gave her great relief. A few weeks later, a similar case presented itself. Things have changed, and more babies arrive to me clothed, but we have a way to go—especially as more and more families are asking for cremations and funerals."

LeighAnne has now dressed more than five thousand babies for their funeral services: from tiny envelope-like pouches for early miscarriages to bigger baby gowns, cardigans, hats, and blankets. She also makes tiny cribs for early pregnancy units. After about sixteen weeks, babies' arms and legs are usually developed enough to be put into these garments, which are made by her team of volunteers—the endearingly named #angelarmy. LeighAnne receives requests all too frequently, and when she was interviewed on the BBC, she received more than one thousand emails the following day. Her charity isn't the only one: another, Heavenly Gowns, relies on a pool of volunteers who transform donated wedding dresses into garments for "angel babies" and supplies them to hospitals, funeral homes, and the bereaved directly.

LeighAnne and I spoke about lost babies who not only have been treated without dignity but also whose memory was encouraged to be entirely forgotten by past hospital practices. A woman contacted her thirty-nine years after her baby died; she still had no idea where it had been taken after its birth. LeighAnne made her an outfit and sent it to her as a keepsake—probably the only tangible register of the baby that she had. I couldn't compare my first miscarriage to this horror, but I did share my hunch with LeighAnne that my twins had been sent from the hospital to their postmortem—and then cremation—naked. Or at least I assume this from the scarring polaroid photographs I have of them.

With my permission, she later sent me two outfits in the mail. I felt overwhelmed when she offered to do this, and unable to speak for my three other lost babies who had disappeared, along with waste. What arrived threw me even more: a tiny pink cotton dress, twenty centimeters long and about ten to fifteen centimeters tapering wide, with minute white stars and pink glitter ribbon detail, with an accompanying pink knitted cardigan, hat, and blanket. The other outfit is a pink sleep bag with a mandarin-style collar and a satin rose flower on the right side, where a tiny chest would have been, with a white knitted cardigan and a blanket.

I had little idea when I first received them how much these tenderly made outfits would become another, profoundly important validation of my babies' earthly existence—nor how much they would make me cry. They sit beside me on a shelf as I write now, and occasionally I find myself feeling them, smelling them, squeezing them, and returning them to their individual cellophane bags with far more care than I do with any of my own clothes. I can now consciously replace any unwanted glimpse in my mind of the haunting photographs—which still happens—with beautiful babies in beautiful clothes.

Just as Claire gave various meanings for her *M* pendant depending on who was asking, and Lucy and Cass lacked the confidence to ask friends to join them at the funeral of their baby, I know that if I were to show my tiny baby outfits to most people, there would be a tricky moment, probably filled with silence. Unlike the passing ritual of a funeral—whether a fire on a beach or a private cremation—keepsakes are another means by which the bereaved convey their love for their unborn. I like to think my two outfits will last as a memorial of sorts, maybe carried forward in time by one of my sons into their own families, along with the stories they have of their almost, sort-of siblings.

ANOTHER, RELATIVELY NEW TO ME, way of imprinting a memory of a miscarried baby is online. One of the biggest changes in the field of memorialization in my lifetime has taken place here, and virtual cemeteries have existed since the internet began to take off in the mid-1990s. Expressing grief online is now a normal thing to do. A Facebook profile of a dead, dear friend of mine remains updated and curated, five years after her death, with comments made about her and to her. Bespoke virtual memorials for miscarried babies also thrive, and the Miscarriage Association is just one portal for this perpetual means of remembering.

At the time of writing, the charity's website curates ten archived "lights of love trees" web pages and forty-one archived "forget-me-not meadows": no longer active for use, they exist in virtual perpetuity. Via placing a light on a tree or the planting of a forget-me-not flower in a meadow, scores of bereaved have created a virtual memorial for their baby, annotated with a message. The current "stars of remembrance" web page is the latest version, where visitors can now create their memorials. It depicts a night sky, constellated with stars—those that glimmer represent a grief. The charity tends to an enormous, little-known accumulation of intangible gravestones that are easy to find, and I encourage you to visit to learn more about what miscarried babies can mean.

I can feel a little overwhelmed when I see this collective gathering of love and loss. I may not have ever known these babies or their parents, but I know that they need to be thought about. I recently visited the stars of remembrance web page and hovered my mouse over a star to reveal its virtual inscription: "In memory of the two children who I never got to meet, who still play and grow older together at the edge of my imagination, who are the missing places at the table, the absent guests at family celebrations, recitals, trips to the park. In the words of the bedtime book I now read to your brother and sister, 'I will love you forever, I will like you for always, as long as I'm living, my baby you'll be. Mummy x.'"

As these words above unquestionably prove, remembered and yearned-for babies are often written into a story of a family left behind. They are frequently named, promised to be thought about, soothed with assurances of meeting their parents again, and reminded of how loved they were and always will be: even if they couldn't be described with an intelligibility discernible to others, because they live at the "edges of imagination." One client of mine kept her virtual memorial for her lost baby readily accessible on her smartphone. She looked at it when feeling vulnerable, such as when family members dismissed her grief or when she remembered the doctor who described her baby as "a bag of cells." Because I knew to ask, she showed it to me with pride.

Tony Walter, the world's only "professor of death studies," at the University of Bath, sees our online memorial culture as the newest chapter in the history of mourning. He knows nothing about the online memorial culture for pregnancy loss though—I asked him—as pregnancy loss hasn't gained any death-study traction. It isn't after all, technically, a death. He notes how both urbanization and industrialization—with their simultaneous medicalization of death—removed us from the visceral and normal realities of death, and thus distanced our relationship with it. However, he sees our recent use of social media and smartphones as having an equally powerful effect in bringing death back, nearer to us and even creating a virtual space where it is no longer the taboo it became. The online world does seem to be a place where the grief and conversation around miscarriage can flow freely, and millions of angel babies can rest in peace.

After a miscarriage at sixteen weeks in 2017, Jessica Zucker, an American psychologist working in the field of pregnancy loss, created the Instagram account ihadamiscarriage to visually document her and other women's experiences. At the time of writing, it has 23,600 followers and curates nearly 800 beautiful images—a breast leaking milk, empty bellies scarred with stretch marks, women with babies, empowering messages of strength. Zucker particularly wanted to address the shame and guilt that women can feel after a miscarriage, and her arresting campaign work (which goes beyond Instagram) illustrates how entwined remembering is with protest too: one of her posts is of an exquisite ten-word poem written by someone named "d.j": "She was not / A chapter. / She was / The whole / Story."

Poems are not a new way of capturing the experience of miscarriage though, even if the platform of Instagram is. I have written about Lady Mary's extraordinary written reflections on her miscarriage from four hundred years ago in my chapter on early loss, and I've lost count of the times I have read probably the best-known miscarriage poem,

"Parliament Hill Fields" by Sylvia Plath. Written in 1961, a week after her miscarriage of her second child-to-be, the poem reflects that this was a time when her child in mind was encouraged to be forgotten, and the taboo of miscarriage had yet to be campaigned for. Nor were there the easy opportunities women have now to publish and share their experiences online. The poem begins in a new year, on a hill, in a park near to her North London home. While she reflects on the "business as usual" nature of the sky above, she talks to her lost baby: "Your absence is inconspicuous; / Nobody can tell what I lack." The rest of the poem is equally moving.

Charities actively encourage the bereaved to publish their stories and poems on their websites, and countless personal stories fill blogs and online chat rooms. These strike me as acts of remembrance and, I have no doubt, act as a source of solace for others. However, the Tommy's online "Book of misCOURAGE" has an explicit campaigning, political edge, offering a virtual "place of support for millions of women to share brave stories of miscarriage. Every story counts. Together, we will create something that can't be ignored, something that helps everyone understand the devastation of miscarriage." Whatever the motive behind storytelling may be, these stories will, I hope, become valuable archives for future social historians too.

It's not always written words that are used to make permanent memorials out of stories of miscarriage and to remember babies by. Creativity in all its forms has been a natural outlet for our grief for centuries—and paintings, photography, sculpture, and music can be healing for the bereaved and a valuable education for everyone. Last year I discovered a new way to think about memorialization practices at a small exhibition in East London's Protein Studios, *Remembering Baby: Life, Loss and Post-Mortem*.

This exhibition explored themes of memory-making after the death of a baby in pregnancy or around birth, the decisions that parents have to make concerning the handling and disposal of their baby's body, and the little-known and developing practice of MRI postmortem procedures. One installation, by artist Justin Wiggan, used an unusual, brilliant way of capturing memory: sound. When I spoke with him he reminded me that our sense of hearing is thought to be our last "working" sense before we die, so it may be that sound memorials could be the most long-lasting in our lifetime.

For this show, he had created two sound pieces of early-life loss. The installation *Lost Boy* concerned memories, and their sounds, of a friend of mine. I knew of her miscarriage fourteen years ago, but the short story version for the installation (displayed in a text beside it) stunned me: "I was a working mum of a two-year-old boy, and was going through a normal, healthy pregnancy . . . Then, from nowhere, I was taken ill, rushed to hospital and told that my tiny baby had died. I went through labour, and said goodbye to my sweet, only just forming, baby boy. He was the size of my hand." Her final paragraph conveys the strength of the ongoing bond she has for her lost son: "At times, the process of being involved in the making of my sound memory has floored me. But this memorial is a powerful and unexpected way to honour my lost boy. There is no gravestone or tree for him, but now there is this, and I am so thankful."

To hear Noah's sound memorial, I climbed into a large mirrored box, sitting in the middle of the exhibition floor. The speakers inside played a piece that represented what had happened before the dreadful event: the rumble of a dishwasher, snatched sounds of children's TV and biscuits coming out of their packet. Then there were noises connoting the time when things went so wrong: a siren, car doors shutting, muffled voices, and beeps familiar to me, from a hospital. Glimpses of what might have been in Noah's future played after: Lego playing, bike rides, and a school assembly. The artist linked these together with birdcalls, which my friend described as "so deftly captur[ing] feelings of helplessness, loss and aching." By writing about this now, I create another memorial for Noah too.

In a previous chapter I wrote about a bereaved father and artist, Foz Foster, who exhibited a seventy-five-foot scroll painting, *Pain Will Not Have the Last Word*, depicting his experience of three miscarriages, as well as of other men's encounters with this kind of loss. His work is part of his ongoing campaign to highlight the oft-ignored experience of partners in miscarriage, but he also spoke of it as a lasting memorial. I encourage you to find the image online— another place where we can join in remembering.

If you haven't seen Frida Kahlo's first painting on metal, *Henry Ford Hospital* (1932), I suggest you search for that too. It shows the artist lying isolated and naked on a hospital bed, with a pool of blood beneath her, after her second miscarriage. Her body is clearly ill at ease in this brutal-looking environment, and a single oversized tear sits on her left cheek. Six objects float around her, connected by red umbilical-like threads that she holds in her left hand: a male fetus (the son she would never have), a snail (signaling the slow horror of loss), an orchid (a gift from her husband), a pelvis (her own was smashed in an accident), and a pink plaster female torso. An ugly, sterilizing machine is tethered to her, and the industrial background of Detroit sets her story in the bleakest of contexts: a patienthood seems to compete with her human, complex story of loss. Kahlo, who died childless, described how her creativity was related to her yearnings for children: "Many things prevented me from fulfilling my desires which everyone considers normal, and to me nothing seemed more natural than to paint what had not been fulfilled."

KAHLO'S SEMINAL PAINTING powerfully conveys how miscarriage—and efforts to remember it—are often a lonely experience, perhaps shared only among kindred mourners of the pregnancy-loss community or specialist medical staff. We have yet to accept that this act of mourning is a fully legitimate one culturally, worthy of the attention we would give other deaths. The truth is, grief after miscarriage still doesn't get the rights that other kinds of grief can claim with greater (although not always straightforward) ease: to be seen, heard, considered, supported, and validated as true. Our efforts to remember can be striven for or, as described by the bereavement scholar K. J. Doka "disenfranchised."

Doka studied the rules that cultures have long constructed around grief and mourning behaviors: how to do it, for how long, and who should do it. People often turn to the

Victorian period for a clear example of when we were notoriously prescriptive about appropriate periods of mourning (for example, a woman would have to mourn her father-in-law longer than her child), as well as the clothes to wear while doing so—such as black dresses, trimmed with crepe silk. But as Doka notes, "grief rules" still linger on in more subtle ways, and many griefs never gain the rights that others unquestionably have.

Doka was particularly interested in the essential role of validation and support—or not—from others, and he noted how both tend to disappear in three situations: where a relationship with the dead is not recognized (such as one with our unborn); where a loss is not recognized (such as that of miscarriage); and where the griever is not recognized (such as if he or she has learning disabilities or is very young). While miscarriage almost always involves the first two scenarios, we know little about how miscarriage is experienced for many marginalized grievers—men, same-sex or nonbinary partners, other family members, teenage mothers and those with learning difficulties or disabilities. We also know very little about the experience of miscarriage among many cultural groups other than white Western secular ones.

ENFRANCHISING THE GRIEF OF MISCARRIAGE, so it acquires the rights it deserves is a political act, as the term suggests. Numerous charities and individuals work hard to make this happen throughout the year, and the growing strength and profile of the UK's Baby Loss Awareness Week—or BLAW—reflects another valuable part of this ongoing effort. This annual event has its roots in campaign work more than thirty years ago in the US: in 1984 the Pregnancy and Infant Loss Center of Minnesota managed to secure a governor's proclamation that October would become Pregnancy and Infant Loss Remembrance Month. Campaign groups in other states then persuaded other states and cities to follow suit. By the late eighties, this movement made it to a federal level, and President Reagan signed a national proclamation in 1988, stating "National observance of Pregnancy and Infant Loss Awareness Month, 1988, offers us the opportunity to increase our understanding of the great tragedy involved in the deaths of unborn and newborn babies." The following October, pregnancy-loss support groups from all over the USA met in Washington, DC, to mark the event.

Linda Layne, in her book *Motherhood Lost*, describes how the bereaved marched with baby blankets embroidered with names, held a service of remembrance and a tree dedication, and made a visit to the late President Kennedy's babies' graves. They called for changes to be made in legislation for sick leave, insurance coverage, income tax deductions, and the disposal of miscarried baby bodies, as well as making a plea for research funding. Other countries have been inspired to follow suit, and similar annual events now take place in the UK, Canada, Australia, Norway, Italy, and Kenya.

In the UK, Baby Loss Awareness Day first happened three months after my first miscarriage in 2002. I can't remember if I was entirely ignorant of the day or felt too raw and frightened to acknowledge it, especially as I was pregnant again by then. By the following year, the day had already expanded to a week of activities, and BLAW has grown in influence and public profile ever since. Its trademark pink-and-blue ribbon pin may sit on a lapel or shirt, in the place where a remembrance poppy might go a week or so later—although the latter is far better known and understood.

BLAW not only involves raising awareness of the impact of baby loss, and of the work of the more than sixty charities involved (in the 2018 event), but as its US founder members also tried to effect, it pushes for the improved care for the bereaved in medical and other settings and the funds for this to happen. The 2017 BLAW saw the launch of the first phase of a new National Bereavement Care Pathway, developed to "improve the quality of bereavement care experienced by parents and families at all stages of pregnancy and baby loss up to 12 months." Additionally, stories were published and broadcast in print and other media, scores of public buildings and landmarks were lit up in pink and blue, memorial services were held, and a debate in the British Parliament discussed the need for improved care and research into miscarriage.

The MP Dr. Philippa Whitford movingly shared her personal experience of pregnancy loss with her political colleagues, teasing out the oft-held misconception that grief increases in relation to a baby's gestational age: "I understand that we are predominantly talking about babies who have been lost later, but that term 'miscarriage' sounds like 'misstep'—like a bump in the road—and by four or five months, particularly once you have had that little ultrasound picture, which you thought was going to be the first of a whole lifetime of photographs, you realise you have already bonded with the bulge that means you need elasticated waistbands and is giving you heartburn or keeping you up at night, or even, a bit later, starting to kick the living daylights out of you at three in the morning . . ."

On the penultimate day of the 2017 BLAW, I joined about twenty other adults, and three infants, on a remembrance walk along London's river Thames, which had been organized by the inspirational Miscarriage Association volunteer Erin, who invited me to her support group. We each held a small heart-shaped battery-powered candle, and some wore T-shirts with the charity's logo. During the two hours of gentle walking, we shared stories of lost babies and lost dreams, good care and bad care, and exchanged ideas of how to spread our net of remembrance further. We walked past the building that houses the UK publisher of this book, a silent contributor to our wishes. A couple of passers-by asked what we were doing, before quickly moving on after we explained; they were interested, perhaps a bit surprised—and, I hope, inspired to think a little bit more.

I was intrigued by a young male fellow walker, barely out of his teens, who was keen to learn as much as possible for a documentary film about miscarriage that he was producing for his undergraduate degree. He knew nothing about the topic—it was a cause close to the director's heart—and was far away from a desire to be a parent (I asked him). I wondered out loud if next year's walk would attract more people like him—those who just wanted to know more. The following night, I lit a candle at 7 p.m., consciously participating in the Wave of Light event that closes BLAW. There's no way of knowing how many other bereaved across the world joined me in doing so, and I confess to an apathy in asking others I know—who hadn't experienced miscarriage—to join me.

WE HAVE A LONG WAY to go before BLAW, and the scores of charities involved in its collective campaign, will no longer be needed. Miscarriage remains a largely ignored experience, with its attendant grief still battling for recognition from the sidelines. I know this from the stories I hear and tell, what I have learned during the process of writing this book, and also because, unwittingly, I have been running an experiment in my kitchen. One effort I made to remember my first miscarriage is testament to my difficult journey of grief and its patchy recognition by many others.

Before leaving the hospital after the birth of my twins, a midwife pressed their four tiny feet into a sponge steeped in pink ink, and then transferred their footprints onto separate white cards. They remain the most important legacy of their beings that I have, and my only tangible link left to the flesh that I had seen on many screens, and felt move inside of me, for many weeks. The unbearable photos we were given hadn't *touched* them, and I had no clothes or blanket that had been in contact with their skin. When we left the hospital that hot summer day, we had already signed away their two bodies for a postmortem, and we had signed them away again for a cremation.

For a couple of years this totem card with their footprints

on it remained in an envelope in a box, in a drawer, under my bed, along with the dreadful photographs and a folded A4 paper from the hospital, which I still haven't read. I guess it records my status as a patient, with details of my admission and discharge, as well as some medical description of what had happened. During that time, I would occasionally blow dust off the box and look at the card, too agonized to linger long, until eventually, about a year after my first son was born, the pain ebbed enough for me to put the card in a frame, and then place the frame on my bedside table. It didn't occur to me to put it on public display in my home, as I had with the plentiful photos of my son.

For a decade, the framed footprints sat beside me as I slept and were directly in the line of the sun that streamed through my window on spring and summer mornings. Very slowly, imperceptibly at first, the sunshine bleached the footprints away. I watched it happen. Year after year, my only link to my babies' soles and twenty teeny toes disappeared before my eyes, yet I was seemingly unable to move the frame. I was frozen—again—by pain, denial, and not-knowing, just as I had been at the time of their births.

The footprints were barely visible when a friend called me in great distress after the miscarriage of her second baby. She needed to talk, and during a conversation over lunch we spoke about how she was going to explain what had happened to her five-year-old daughter, as well as how she was determined to mark the death of her second child-to-be. She wondered about holding a private funeral and spoke passionately about her commitment to the idea of keeping the memory of her baby alive.

For some reason, that conversation touched a nerve, even though it was far from a new topic for me. She made me realize how hypocritical I had been—understandably, forgivably, but even so. I have long campaigned for all of us to talk more openly about miscarriage and urged others to think about and unhush the experience for the sake of those who suffer. But while doing so, I had kept my only real link to my babies hidden, and then almost vanished them away. I had also assumed that I talked about my miscarriages freely, but I realized it was only really among friends who I knew had experienced a grief like mine, or with people who worked in the field of pregnancy loss. My friend inspired me to take action, and she was able to help me in a practical way too.

A photographer by profession, she introduced me to a colleague of hers who, with digital wizardry, restored the footprints to their original pink and exquisitely detailed state. I could see again how Florence's left foot was pushed down too hard, so its arch can't be discerned, and was reminded of my regret at my decision not to hold it—or the other three feet, legs, arms, and bodies. I bought a bigger, bolder frame to put the image in and hung it at the head of my kitchen table, next to a map of quirky English place-names, well away from the bleaching effect of the sun.

These feet provoke far less conversation than their neighboring picture ever has, or indeed the print of Tracey Emin's naked running body from behind, hung on the opposite wall. Not one visitor to my kitchen has stopped to read the inscriptions under each pair of perfect pink feet: "Matilda 31.07.02, Florence 1.08.02"—or asked anything about them. Maybe it's because people assume these prints are of my sons' feet, maybe they just don't notice them, but I suspect it's more to do with a reluctance to embark on a conversation that has no well-worn trajectory.

While these ghost family members may still struggle to inhabit other people's minds, placing them in the thick of my family life made the writing of this book possible. It aims to honor the memories of not only my three other babies whose feet we couldn't press into ink but also the millions of other lost babies who continue to be a part of millions of others' lives—whether you know personally of them or not.

Epilogue

As I was coming to the end of writing this book, a timely request from a friend over dinner helped me along. She wanted my advice: a colleague in her team at work had just told her, by email, that her twelve-week scan had revealed that her "baby" (her colleague's words) had died a couple of weeks previously. She needed to have surgery and wouldn't be in the office for a week or so. My friend, who knew nothing of the pregnancy, was clearly concerned by the news, but she had stalled at the next step: knowing *how to think* about an appropriate response—and therefore to know what to do or to say.

Knowing my friend very well, this topic of conversation felt like progress to me—while she had acknowledged my first miscarriage with kindness, she had seemed baffled when my subsequent miscarriages, at earlier gestations, hit me badly. She was far from alone in her response and had talked to me about her one early miscarriage as an unfortunate but forgettable thing that had happened. I like to think

I had an influence on how her thinking and empathy broadened over time, but whatever the reasons, she had come to know that her colleague's news deserved more thought than she may have previously given it. I will come back to my response.

My friend's shift in view is indicative of a larger, more-than-welcome cultural one: we *are* considering the impact of miscarriage more than ever before. Or rather, maybe we are considering it no more than before, but are more willing to broach the subject. Years of campaign work from the bereaved and growing numbers of pregnancy-loss charities, along with more confident storytelling in the media, have all contributed to this. The online world has also made this advocacy easier, enabling both individual and collective efforts to confront rather than avoid this especially thorny topic. But just as these voices help educate others, and move thinking along, they collectively remind us that there is still great room for improvement: both within the medical arena and beyond it.

The medical care of miscarriage matters greatly because it can become an inextricable part of the miscarriage experience and our lasting memories of it. Despite having received some wonderful care in hospitals, it's the bad care that still stings: the doctor who thought I was being histrionic for not wanting to push my dead babies out of me; the anesthetist who became bored of my tears before my surgery; and whoever it was who threw my baby away without my consent. Through ignorance or lack of training or who knows what, these episodes of mis-attuned care aren't isolated anecdotes either: they pile up on the, sadly, still-growing heap of similar versions.

Years on from my own experiences, and despite many more good practices and protocols in place, I continue to hear plenty of stories that echo mine. Women still run the risk of hearing their miscarried babies described as "mucky bits" by a health-care staff member or of having their baby who has been removed by surgery put in the wrong container and then lost. Women are still sent home to miscarry without adequate information about their pain or what will leave their womb or the potential for breast milk being produced. Many aren't informed about how they can preserve their baby for a funeral ritual that they may well desire, or at least want to know the option for, but feel coy about. Partners and other family members may well grieve too yet are overlooked while being relied on to plug the gaps of care. And many couples will go on to have another pregnancy riddled with anxiety or even more serious mental health problems, without adequate emotional support or understanding. None of this seems right to me, but I am hopeful.

I write at a potentially exciting time for miscarriage care in the UK. There is no doubt that exemplary care does already exist, however there is a woeful variability in standards. But there is a potential antidote to this in a pilot project, launched in late 2017: the National Bereavement Care Pathway, which builds on years of campaign work and changes in practice that have been made to date. This sets out a number of guidelines, co-devised by baby-loss charities and professional bodies, for best practice for all professionals delivering bereavement care for five bereavement experiences: miscarriage, ectopic pregnancies and molar pregnancies, the ending of a pregnancy after a prenatal diagnosis, stillbirth, neonatal death, and the sudden unexpected death in infancy.

This pathway structure is also an important reflection of joined-up thinking: a miscarrying woman under medical care may come across a number of health-care professionals and may have to make a number of difficult decisions for the care of her body and her baby's body. While labor wards and early pregnancy units generally have the best training and experience when it comes to miscarriage care, a woman may end up being treated in other medical contexts where this tends to be less reliable: accident and emergency departments, GP practices, sonography rooms, or surgery and gynecology wards.

The new guidance for miscarriage and ectopic and molar pregnancy care sets out comprehensive recommendations for all staff who deal with a patient (a woman, a mother) losing a baby—or pregnancy—under their care, as well as her partner and family. Topics include the use of language, compassionate communication, the experiences of both early and late miscarriage, delivering difficult news, making memories, decisions around postmortems, certification of babies that existed but aren't stillborn, funerals, and sensitive disposal, as well as emotional care after loss and the importance of support for staff involved.

Unlike those who know less about the potentially broad and diverse experience of miscarriage, when it comes to parity of good care, the contributors of the NBCP do not seem to get hung up on the differences between a baby lost before twenty-four weeks and one who dies later on or at or after birth. This is testament to the possibility that the grief for a baby held more in mind than body may be as worthy of institutional consideration and support as one born near or at full term.

What is also encouraging is that the pilot rolls out (as I write, thirty-two NHS Trusts are involved) because of the influence of the All-Party Parliamentary Group on Baby Loss, founded in early 2016 by four MPs with personal experiences of bereavement. This group continues to pressure Parliament (and devolved administrations of Scotland, Wales, and Northern Ireland—at the moment, the NBCP applies to England alone) to help prevent and reduce deaths of babies of all gestations, as well as to improve the care that the bereaved receive. I have sat in a House of Commons committee room at one of their meetings, buoyed by their obvious commitment. In early 2018, 106,000 pounds of government funding was announced to further its work for a year—we need more, of course.

As this unprecedented political work reiterates, we need to keep up the pressure to prioritize the allocation of resources that enable such good practice to percolate further through the health-care system. This includes funding for training budgets for staff, the provision of resources and emotional support, and the research to support evidence-based practice. Encouraged as I am by the fact that improved care for miscarriage is on important agendas, I also write in times of austerity and political upheaval, with the NHS under tremendous strain. Any or all of these factors could easily sabotage the universality and comprehensive nature of these hoped-for changes.

This hard-earned consciousness raising—of which the NBCP is a contemporary leading example—is only one part of the ongoing effort to improve the care for miscarriage. As so many couples discover in the wake of their heartache, miscarriage is common yet generally little understood, and this lack of knowledge compounds the grief of so many bereaved. Many are left frustrated and angered by a medical paradigm that can offer so much to so many, yet so little to a couple who just want to make a baby who lives. But I'm cautiously hopeful about this too: research into the causation and prevention of miscarriage now rides a wave of interest and funding that we have never seen before.

In April 2016, Tommy's National Centre for Miscarriage Research was inaugurated as the largest of its kind in Europe. Bringing together already established international expertise in the field, it is poised as the vanguard of collaborative work to explore four key research enquiries: Why does miscarriage happen? Will it happen again? Can it be prevented? Can we better understand the lived experience of those who suffer? When the media reported on this center's launch, countless hearts were lifted—not only because of the prospect of future prevention and treatment, but also because miscarriage was being reported on in the first place.

At the time of writing, Tommy's undertakes and supports a broad portfolio of research. Some explores potential causes with a view to developing diagnostic tests—such as the role of sperm DNA fragmentation, among various genetic studies. Other work includes pursuing a better understanding of the role of the immune system in women who have recurrent miscarriages, as well as the potential use of a drug originally designed for diabetes to help prevent further losses. The psychological effects of miscarriage are also being studied, with a view to devising, and tailoring, the best emotional care for those in distress. It is hoped that this unprecedented network of researchers from a number of disciplines will be better able to pool their expertise to both identify key research questions and design quality clinical trials to address them.

Around the time that the Tommy's center opened, another encouraging collaboration emerged: the Miscarriage Priority Setting Partnership, which brings together professionals concerned with miscarriage care and those directly affected by miscarriage to hear their views about priorities for research—rather than relying on those set by researchers or even the pharmaceutical industry. While some of the questions that have been captured by participants are already being addressed by researchers, it's encouraging to think that further research may be driven by those who have experienced miscarriage firsthand.

But the truth remains that for many more years to come, miscarriages will happen, frequently, to many women and couples. We have to bide our time when it comes to upping the chance of prevention or treatment: research trials take years to be conducted and analyzed and their results then disseminated and acted on. As Professor Arri Coomarasamy, the director of the Tommy's National Centre for Miscarriage

Research, said to me, "we are at the tip of the iceberg" in our research endeavors, and any more breakthroughs in understanding the causes of miscarriage are likely to be incremental, as they have been so far.

While this heartening work goes on, there is much more that we can do outside of hospital and laboratory buildings. We are all capable of making the experience of miscarriage for the bereaved more bearable—as my friend mentioned at the start of this Epilogue thought that she ought to for her colleague. Generally reluctant to give anyone advice—the therapist in me is tenacious—I was deliberately playful with her in my response that night over dinner. I suggested a number of questions—not necessarily to be asked—with the intention of sparking new thinking. I knew the questions were mainly inappropriate in the context she faced, but I also knew it was highly likely that my friend would encounter miscarriage again and I wanted to prepare her.

I said something like, "Think about these questions: How did your miscarriage begin? How long did it take? Were you at home, or did you go to the hospital? Was the pain bearable? Did you lose lots of blood? Were you looked after okay? Did you see your baby on a screen? Did you hold your baby? Did you know if it was a boy or girl? Did you have a sense of whether it was a boy or girl? Did you name him or her? Did you get to wash your baby or dress him or her? How long did you have to be with your baby? Did he or she look like one of you? Did you take photos? Do you have any keepsakes? Do you know why your baby died? Will you have a postmortem? Will you have a funeral? Did your milk come in? What will you do with your milk? How is your partner? . . ."

I didn't mean to suggest that she conduct an interrogation, but I could see as I spoke how I had inspired something in my friend: her eyes widened, her jaw dropped, and she began to nod. I seemed to have lifted the lid off a container she—with the help of many others—had sealed shut. I don't know how she responded to her colleague, but I found out later how our conversation had been thought provoking and that she had shared its theme with others. In short, she thought more, and she thought differently—with greater curiosity, empathy, and compassion. My hope is that this book does this for you too.

Acknowledgments

I asked many people to help me with this book and I was consistently met with encouragement and generosity, as opposed to mere agreement. Both Katie Bond and Mary Mount put the initial wind in my sails to transfer my inchoate ramblings onto paper, and without their efforts, I wouldn't have captured the attention of my indomitable agent, Carrie Plitt. As a debut author with a topic that was not going to be a straightforward sell, Carrie had a tough job ahead of her, and I remain in awe of her persuasive powers.

I think the four most beautiful consecutive words I use are *The Brink of Being,* and these I owe to the brilliant poet Julia Copus. Her permission to use them, from her exquisite poem *Ghost,* remains a treasured gift. I knew of Julia's work through the super-human endeavors of Jessica Hepburn, who continues to raise the profile of the pain and injustices of infertility, and its treatment, in creative and unprecedented ways. Without Jessica, I also wouldn't have met

Dr. Isabelle Davis, Jody Day, or Dr. Robin Hadley—all of whom pushed my thinking in welcome directions.

More thanks to Dr. Jackie Ross, Dr. Sheelagh McGuinness, Helen Williams, and Dr. Karolina Kuberska. Helen made my meeting with Dr. Ari Coomarasamy happen. I am grateful for his valuable time, but also his obvious compassion and championship of my efforts. One bonus of my past Trusteeship at the Miscarriage Association is an ongoing friendship with Dr. Nicola Davies, who hosted me on the hottest day in her garden and introduced me to the phenomenal Morag Kinghorn. Penny Kerry, another M.A. stalwart, managed to find the time to read a very early draft of my manuscript without giving up, or being too rude about it.

My thanks to Dr. Tanya Cassidy and Gillian Weaver for fascinating conversations about the politics and donation of breast milk, and my walk on a Pembrokeshire beach with Dr. Natalie Shenker, discussing the same, remains one of my research highlights. LeighAnne Wright gave me much of her precious time, and along with the Superintendent of Golders Green Cemetery and the staff of Wigley & Sons Funeral Directors, taught me more about the pragmatics of human death than I ever knew before. I am so grateful to Dr. Sarah Bailey—for plenty of her time, valuable thoughts, and inspiring work with her patients.

My meeting with Zoe Chamberlain sowed many useful seeds and other fascinating conversations with Tracey Sainsbury, Erika Barbra-Muller, Dr. Matt Prior, Professor Helen King, Mr. Charles Wright, Dr. Sarah Bailey, and Rachel Hayden sowed even more that I reluctantly had to leave behind. Across the Atlantic, and battling with time zones, I am very grateful to Patti Budnik from SHARE and Cathi Lammert from PLIDA.

A special thanks to Erica Stewart from Sands, whose infectious energy during our afternoon together lingered with me awhile. Erin Sharkey is a legend, and I'm proud to now be her friend and humbled to be taking her place with Erica Charlton at the monthly support group they run on behalf of the Miscarriage Association. Erin and Erica join Cherie Raphael at UCLH as just three of countless unsung heroes amongst hospital staff, and charity volunteers, who support bereaved parents every day.

My friends Anya Sizer, Helen Moyes, Alison Wright, Claire Usiskin, Carrie O'Grady, Angela Norris, Tara Darby, Sophie Hare, and Anna Wraith nudged me in ways they'll never know.

Of course none of these people would need to be thanked if it weren't for the risks taken, and patience suffered, by Sarah Savitt at Virago, and Lindsey Schwoeri and Gretchen Schmidt at Penguin USA, along with their colleagues. I know how lucky I am to have such close attention paid to my text, even at times that were more convenient to me than for them.

This book also wouldn't exist without the unwavering help over many years from Ruth Bender Atik at the Miscarriage Association. Ruth has put up with me in various guises since our first conversation soon after Matilda and Florence were buried. How she carved time out of an impossibly busy schedule to read—and comment on—both my proposal and draft manuscript still baffles me, but without either of these "rubber stamps," I wouldn't have had the confidence to go any further.

Nor could I have written this book without the women I have spoken with over the years. I remain enormously grateful to those who entrust me with their stories, and for deepening my understanding of the miscarriage experience, along with the human condition.

But my biggest thanks is to David. His relentless belief in me, and his uncomplaining willingness to pick up more than his fair share of domestic responsibilities during the intense period of writing, paved my way. Also, as father to all of our babies, I want to acknowledge his unflinching generosity in letting me share his private life too. Without David, I couldn't have done, nor wouldn't do, anything of use at all.

Notes

Introduction

xix is often quoted to affect: The Miscarriage Association and Tommy's suggest one in four pregnancies ends in miscarriage, while research papers are inconsistent due to the difficulty of diagnosing true incidence, as many miscarriages go unnoticed or unreported. Most studies report that around 1 in 5 clinical pregnancies will miscarry (before 24 weeks), yet others looking at conception and early pregnancy have reported loss rates of up to 1 in 3. The commonly quoted "one in four" seems to composite these findings as in N. Maconochie et al. "Risk factors for first trimester miscarriage—results from a UK-population-based case–control study." *BJOG: An International Journal of Obstetrics & Gynaecology.* Feb 1, 2007;114(2):170–86.

xix a recent US national survey: Jonah Bardos et al., "A National Survey on Public Perceptions of Miscarriage," *Obstetrics & Gynecology* 125, no. 6 (June 2015): 1313–20. In the US, the upper limit of miscarriage is defined at twenty weeks (with state differences according to weight).

xix Another estimate for the UK suggested: https://www.tommys.org/our -organisation/charity-research/pregnancy-statistics.

xx A report from the Office for National Statistics: "Births in England and Wales: 2015," Office for National Statistics, July 13, 2016, https://www .ons.gov.uk/peoplepopulationandcommunity/birthsdeathsandmarriages /livebirths/bulletins/birthsummarytablesenglandandwales/2015.

xxv most miscarriages happen early on: The research papers quote differing statistics: with either 1 percent happening after twelve weeks' gestation as in Allen J. Wilcox et al., "Incidence of Early Loss of Pregnancy," *The New England Journal of Medicine* 319, no. 4 (July 28, 1988): 189–194; or 4 percent happening between twelve and twenty-two weeks as quoted in Elisabeth Clare Larsen et al., "New Insights into Mechanisms behind Miscarriage," *BMC*

Medicine 11, no. 1 (2013): 154. To confuse things more, Tommy's suggests 85 percent of pregnancies end before twelve weeks: https://www.tommys .org/pregnancy-information/im-pregnant/early-days-pregnancy/how -common-miscarriage.

xxvi essential changes are beginning: Dr. Susie Kilshaw, principal research fellow at University College London, has researched the impact of miscarriage in Qatar and tells me of other fascinating anthropological studies such as Erica van der Sijpt's work in Romania and Cameroon. Dr. Kilshaw is co-editing (with Katie Borg) a volume of international studies as I write: *Negotiating Miscarriage: A Social, Medical and Conceptual Problem,* to be published by Berghahn Books. I also see research literature exploring the experience of miscarriage coming from Iran, Taiwan, Japan, and Hong Kong.

xxvii in the context of pregnancy loss: Linda L. Layne, *Motherhood Lost: A Feminist Account of Pregnancy Loss in America* (London: Routledge, 2003), 240.

Chapter One: A Child in Mind

6 the presence of the hormone: HCG is produced by the syncytiotrophoblast—the beginnings of the placenta.

7 "For us, their voices are silent": Suszannah Lipscomb, "Silenced Voices," *The Times Literary Supplement* (December 5, 2017).

9 Some vivid depictions of pregnancy: Cathy McClive and Helen King, "When Is a Foetus not a Foetus? Diagnosing False Conceptions in Early Modern France," in *L'embryon humain à travers l'histoire: Images, savoirs et rites,* ed. Véronique Dasen (Gollion: Infolio, 2007): 223–238.

9 animated enough to be sensed: Barbara Duden, *The Woman Beneath the Skin: A Doctor's Patients in Eighteenth-Century Germany,* trans. Thomas Dunlap (Cambridge: Harvard University Press, 1998).

9 "'a foul mass of flesh'": Eve Keller, "Embryonic Individuals: The Rhetoric of Seventeenth-Century Embryology and the Construction of Early-Modern Identity," *Eighteenth-Century Studies* 33, no. 3 (Spring 2000): 328.

10 testing became mainstream: Jesse Olszynko-Gryn, "The Feminist Appropriation of Pregnancy Testing in 1970s Britain," *Women's History Review* (2017): 1–26.

11 visual message of apparent autonomy: Yet it can be used for political purposes too, as such imagery is also used by pro-life movements to shackle women's choice.

12 "Your Baby at Week 6": https://www.whattoexpect.com/pregnancy/week -by-week/week-6.aspx.

12 The author Rachel Cusk: Rachel Cusk, *A Life's Work: On Becoming a Mother* (New York: Picador, 2015), 21.

13–14 the spirit-child can then enter: Janet L. Sha, *Mothers of Thyme: Customs and Rituals of Infertility and Miscarriage* (Ann Arbor, Lida Rose Press, 1990), 65.

15 the traditional practice of Taegyo: N.I. Noh and H.A. Yeom, "Development of the Korean Paternal-Fetal Attachment Scale (K-PAFAS)," *Asian Nursing Research* (2017).

15 "I have been tagged": Cusk, *A Life's Work*, 31. And for more on prescriptions on pregnant women: Deborah Lupton, "'Precious cargo': Foetal Subjects, Risk and Reproductive Citizenship," *Critical Public Health* 22, no. 3 (2012): 329–40.

16 "Your Baby at Week 9": https://www.whattoexpect.com/pregnancy/week -by-week/week-9.aspx.

17 may have strenthened her bond: Nathan Stormer, "Seeing the Fetus: The Role of Technology and Image in the Maternal-Fetal Relationship," *JAMA* 289, no. 13 (April 2, 2003): 1700.

19 "every mother mourned": John H. Kennell, Howard Slyter, and Marshall H. Klaus, "The Mourning Response of Parents to the Death of a Newborn Infant," *The New England Journal of Medicine* 283, no. 7 (1970): 344–49.

19 "magnified into a catastrophe": Stanford Bourne and Emanuel Lewis, "Perinatal Bereavement," *The BMJ* 302, no. 6786 (May 18, 1991): 1167.

19 "the disturbed doctor-patient relationship": Stanford Bourne, "The Psychological Effects of Stillbirths on Women and Their Doctors," *The Journal of the Royal College of General Practitioners,* 16(2), (1968), 103.

20 "professional deafness": Stanford Bourne, "The Psychological Effects of Stillbirths on Women and Their Doctors," *The Journal of the Royal College of General Practitioners,* 16(2), (1968), 103.

22 scanned the brains: Elseline Hoekzema et al., "Pregnancy Leads to Long-Lasting Changes in Human Brain Structure," *Nature Neuroscience* 20, no. 2 (2017): 287–296.

25 No hard conclusions from the studies: Jeanne L. Alhusen, "A Literature Update on Maternal-Fetal Attachment," *Journal of Obstetric, Gynecologic & Neonatal Nursing* 37, no. 3 (2008): 315–328.

27 expecting a baby that never arrived: I owe many thanks to Dr. Isabel Davis for my conversation about all of this.

27 her case as one of pseudocyesis: Where twelve women who "believed they were pregnant" were described.

28 phenomenon is scarcely recorded: Stephanie J. Campos and Denise Link, "Pseudocyesis," *The Journal for Nurse Practitioners* 12, no. 6 (June 2016): 390–94 quotes an incidence of one to six out of twenty-two thousand births in the Western world.

28 cultural and familial pressure: Mary V. Seeman, "Pseudocyesis, Delusional Pregnancy, and Psychosis: The Birth of a Delusion," *World Journal of Clinical Cases* 2, no. 8 (August 16, 2014): 338. I also spoke with an obstetrician who, during fifty years of practice in London, never encountered a case of pseudocyesis. He did however meet it in Zululand, South Africa, in the late 1960s when women spent little time with their husbands during the year—most had gone to earn money in mining towns far away. There was tremendous pressure to conceive when they were briefly together. Perhaps these women's strong desire, combined with a cultural expectation of motherhood, sparked their strong belief that they had a growing baby inside them. Bellies would swell, sickness would be endured.

29 molar or an ectopic pregnancy: It could also be said that the unpleasantly named "blighted ovum" challenges "normal" conception too. Here an embryo fails to grow at all or begins to grow shortly before stopping. A pregnancy sac continues to grow regardless though.

31 In Jessica's case: Jessica Rüb, "Dear Mother with the Crying Baby," Miscarriage Association, http://www.miscarriageassociation.org.uk/story/dear-mother-crying-baby/.

32 more than 8 million IVF babies: European Society of Human Reproduction and Embryology, "More than 8 million Babies Born from IVF Since the World's First in 1978," ScienceDaily, https://www.sciencedaily.com/releases/2018/07/180703084127.htm.

32 "Our Miracle called Louise": The Weekly News, published in Dundee, Scotland. As viewed on https://www.louisejoybrown.com/book/.

36 This placement is deliberately done: David Ellison and Isabel Karpin, "Embryo Disposition and the New Death Scene," *Cultural Studies Review* 17, no. 1 (2011): 81.

Chapter Two: Derailed

39 happen in the first trimester: Please see note p. xxv Introduction.

40 pointing to an undetectable phenomenon: Elisabeth Clare Larsen et al., "New Insights into Mechanisms behind Miscarriage," *BMC Medicine* 11, no. 1 (2013): 154.

43 contemporary school curriculum: The recently formed Fertility Education Initiative, https://britishfertilitysociety.org.uk/fei/.

43 popular pregnancy bible: Heidi Murkoff, *What to Expect When You're Expecting* (New York: Workman Publishing, 2016). Now in its fifth edition; I think I had the second.

45 drowned out by protocols and procedures: In the UK, the Royal College of Obstetricians & Gynaecologists' Women's Voices initiative is one effort to counter this.

46 she would avoid a death sentence: Cathy McClive, "The Hidden Truths of the Belly: The Uncertainties of Pregnancy in Early Modern Europe: Society for the Social History of Medicine Student Prize Essay 1999, Runner-up," *Social History of Medicine* 15, no. 2 (August 1, 2002): 209–27. This looks, in particular, at cases of "pleading the belly."

49 Around 137,000 women in England: NICE 2010 Pain and Bleeding in Early Pregnancy: Final Scope. This figure refers to "secondary care" usually delivered in a hospital or clinic, www.nice.org.uk.

49 This lack of clear data: There have been attempts to unify early pregnancy taxonomy and terminology. Time will tell if they take off.

50 health-care professionals in emergency departments: As quoted in Kate MacWilliams et al., "Understanding the Experience of Miscarriage in the Emergency Department," *Journal of Emergency Nursing* 42, no. 6 (November 2016): 504–12.

51 better education around miscarriage care: This is also addressed in the 2017 launch of the National Bereavement Care Pathway in England.

51 a potential "emotional emergency": http://www.nationalperinatal.org /position. And see the more recent: Anita Catlin, "Interdisciplinary Guidelines for Care of Women Presenting to the Emergency Department with Pregnancy Loss," *MCN: The American Journal of Maternal/Child Nursing* 43, no. 1 (January/February 2018): 13–18.

51 marginalized, ignored, or even forgotten: MacWilliams et al., "Understanding the Experience of Miscarriage," 504–12.

51 the whole visceral truth: The Miscarriage Support Auckland website has a refreshingly honest account of a possible early miscarriage, https://www .miscarriagesupport.org.nz.

52 what a miscarriage will mean: Debra Betts, Hannah G. Dahlen, and Caroline A. Smith, "A Search for Hope and Understanding: An Analysis of Threatened Miscarriage Internet Forums," *Midwifery* 30, no. 6 (January 2013): 650–6.

53 clinical guidance in the UK: https://cks.nice.org.uk/miscarriage. Accessible in the UK.

55 "poore despised Creature": Raymond A. Anselment, "'A Heart Terrifying Sorrow': An Occasional Piece on Poetry of Miscarriage," *Papers on Language and Literature* 33, no. 1 (1997): 13.

55 baby on YouTube: https://www.youtube.com/watch?v=3ytcVF2ll8E.

56 half a million visitors: February 2018. I notice how this number of viewers leaps up each time I reviewed my text.

57 at the bedside of miscarrying women: Shannon K. Withycombe, "From Women's Expectations to Scientific Specimens: The Fate of Miscarriage Materials in Nineteenth-Century America," *Social History of Medicine* 28, no. 2 (May 1, 2015): 245–62.

59 some serious chromosomal problems: The majority of sporadic losses before ten weeks' gestation result from random numeric chromosomal errors: trisomy, monosomy, and polyploidy. Kate Louise McBride and James Patrick Beirne, "Recurrent Miscarriage," *InnovAiT* 7, no. 1 (January 1, 2014): 25–34.

59 Explanations when they *are* given: Ana V. Nikčević and Kypros H. Nicolaides, "Search for Meaning, Finding Meaning and Adjustment in Women Following Miscarriage: A Longitudinal Study," *Psychology & Health* 29, no. 1 (2014): 50–63.

60 **"What he doth spy?":** Sara Read, "'Thanksgiving After Twice Miscarrying': Divine Will and Miscarriage in Early Modern England," *Women's History* 2, no. 5 (2016): 11–15.

61 **a pregnant Roman woman:** Joan Stivala, "Malaria and Miscarriage in Ancient Rome," *Canadian Bulletin of Medical History* 32, no. 1 (Spring 2015): 143–61.

61 **American physician Dr. Joseph DeLee:** Referenced in Shulamit Reinharz, "Controlling Women's Lives: A Cross-Cultural Interpretation of Miscarriage Accounts," *Research in the Sociology of Health Care* 7 (1988): 3–37.

61 **women blamed their own actions:** Rebecca K. Simmons et al., "Experience of Miscarriage in the UK: Qualitative Findings from the National Women's Health Study," *Social Science & Medicine* 63, no. 7 (October 2006): 1934–46.

62 **generally accepted that women shouldn't:** Raj Rai and Lesley Regan, "Recurrent Miscarriage," *The Lancet* 368, no. 9535 (August 12, 2006): 601–11.

62 **Recent guidance about the treatment:** *Recurrent Pregnancy Loss: Guideline of the European Society of Human Reproduction and Embryology*, 2017, https://www.eshre.eu/Guidelines-and-Legal/Guidelines/Recurrent-pregnancy-loss.aspx.

62 **Advanced maternal age:** E. de la Rochebrochard, and P. Thonneau, "Paternal Age and Maternal Age Are Risk Factors for Miscarriage; Results of a Multicentre European Study," *Human Reproduction*, 17 no. 6 (2002):1649–56.

62 **While the risk of miscarriage:** Anne-Marie Nybo Andersen et al., "Maternal Age and Fetal Loss: Population Based Register Linkage Study," *BMJ* 320, no. 7251 (2000): 1708–12.

63 **have been linked to miscarriage:** N. Maconochie et al., "Risk Factors for First Trimester Miscarriage—Results from a UK-Population-Based Case–Control Study," *BJOG: An International Journal of Obstetrics & Gynaecology* 114, no. 2 (2006): 170–186. The authors state that findings in relation to trauma, major life events during pregnancy, and stressful employment "require confirmation."

63 **"The impact of stress":** The European Society of Human Reproduction and Embryology developed a clinical practice guideline, published November 2017, for *Recurrent Pregnancy Loss*, 25.

63 **the NHS website:** http://www.nhs.uk/Conditions/Miscarriage/Pages/Causes.aspx.

63 **the effects of stress:** Jacky Boivin and Sofia Gameiro, "Evolution of Psychology and Counseling in Infertility," *Fertility and Sterility* 104, no. 2 (August 2015): 251–59.

64 **a mother's stress:** Fan Qu et al., "The Association between Psychological Stress and Miscarriage: A Systematic Review and Meta-Analysis," *Scientific Reports* 7, no. 1 (December 2017).

64 **a woman's unresolved psychological issues:** Quoted in Irving G. Leon, *When a Baby Dies: Psychotherapy for Pregnancy and Newborn Loss* (New Haven: Yale University Press, 1992), 49.

68 a particularly tricky setting: Mary Ann Hazen, "Grief and the Workplace," *Academy of Management Perspectives* 22, no. 3 (2008): 78–86; Mary Ann Hazen, "Societal and Workplace Responses to Perinatal Loss: Disenfranchised Grief or Healing Connection," *Human Relations* 56, no. 2 (2003): 147–66.

68 As one research paper concludes: Neil Thompson and Dale A. Lund, *Loss, Grief, and Trauma in the Workplace* (London: Routledge, 2017). First published 2009 by Baywood Publishing Company.

71 wanted to see my baby: At least one hospital in the UK now offers to give women and couples scan photos of early miscarried babies: Joanna Lovell, "Women Who Suffer Early Miscarriages Can Now Get a Scan Picture of Their Baby to Keep," Hull Live, updated February 27, 2018, https://www.hulldailymail.co.uk/news/hull-east-yorkshire-news/women-who-suffer-early-miscarriages-1270128.

Chapter Three: A Conspicuous Absence

79 For sale: baby shoes: The only traceable source of this famous flash fiction can be found in "a play based on the legendary lives of Ernest Hemingway," *Papa,* by John deGroot, Boise State Univ Bookstore, 1989.

79 It is generally accepted: The statistics on early/late miscarriage aren't unified among researchers. Tommy's states on its website that three in four miscarriages happen during the first twelve weeks, https://www.tommys.org/our-organisation/charity-research/pregnancy-statistics/miscarriage, but other papers quote differently—e.g., only 1 percent of miscarriages happen after twelve weeks: Allen J. Wilcox et al., "Incidence of Early Loss of Pregnancy," *The New England Journal of Medicine* 319, no. 4 (July 28, 1988): 189–194. Another recent study conducted in a large Dublin maternity hospital reported a rate of secondary-trimester pregnancy loss as 0.8 percent: Sarah Cullen et al., "Exploring Parents' Experiences of Care in an Irish Hospital Following Second-Trimester Miscarriage," *BJM: British Journal of Midwifery* 25, no. 2 (2017).

83 Statistics about lesbian motherhood: Susan Golombok et al., "Children With Lesbian Parents: A Community Study," *Developmental Psychology* 39, no. 1 (2003): 20.

83 same-sex parents: New Family Social, http://www.newfamilysocial.org.uk/resources/research/statistics/.

83 same-sex couples had children: As quoted in Elizabeth Peel, "Pregnancy Loss in Lesbian and Bisexual Women: An Online Survey of Experiences," *Human Reproduction* 25, no. 3 (March 2010): 721–7; first published online December 19, 2009.

83 lesbian partner's experience: Elizabeth Peel and Ruth Cain, "'Silent' Miscarriage and Deafening Heteronormativity: A British Experiential and Critical Feminist Account," in *Understanding Reproductive Loss: Perspectives on Life, Death and Fertility*, eds. Sarah Earle, Carol Komaromy, and Linda

Layne (London: Routledge, 2016), 79–92; first published 2012 by Ashgate Publishing. "Pervasive heteronormativity doubly marginalises the experiences of lesbians—and women otherwise located outside the realm of heterosexual relationships."

83 **One feminist researcher:** Lisa Cosgrove, "The Aftermath of Pregnancy Loss: A Feminist Critique of the Literature and Implications for Treatment," *Women & Therapy* 27, no. 3–4 (March 2004): 113–14.

86 **closely monitored for pregnancy signs:** Laura Gowing, "Secret Births and Infanticide in Seventeenth-Century England," *Past & Present* 156 (August 1997): 87–115.

89 **Maternity units in England:** A 2016 survey by Sands showed 63% of 62 Trusts and Health Boards had a specialist bereavement room in each maternity unit. (Audit of bereavement care provision in the UK maternity units)

89 **out of earshot:** Only 41 percent of units surveyed could claim this.

91 **midwives' experiences of caring:** Reem Alghamdi and Patricia Jarrett, "Experiences of Student Midwives in the Care of Women with Perinatal Loss: A Qualitative Descriptive Study," *BJM: British Journal of Midwifery* 24, no. 10 (2016): 715–22.

95 **a discomfiting metaphor:** Emanuel Lewis, "Mourning by the Family After a Stillbirth or Neonatal Death," *Archives of Disease in Childhood* 54, no. 4 (1979): 303–6.

96 **language of "monstrosity":** Cathy McClive, "The Hidden Truths of the Belly: The Uncertainties of Pregnancy in Early Modern Europe: Society for the Social History of Medicine Student Prize Essay 1999, Runner-up," *Social History of Medicine* 15, no. 2 (August 1, 2002): 209–27.

96 **"pecking order" of gestational loss:** Alice Lovell, "Some Questions of Identity: Late Miscarriage, Stillbirth and Perinatal Loss," *Social Science & Medicine* 17, no. 11 (1983): 755–61.

98 **led NICE to supplement:** Maura O'Malley, "NICE Clarifies Its Stillbirth Guidelines," The Royal College of Midwives, posted June 25, 2010, https://www.rcm.org.uk/news-views-and-analysis/news/nice-clarifies-its-stillbirth-guidelines. This was reiterated by NICE in a 2014 update of their *Antenatal and Postnatal Mental Health: Clinical Management and Service Guidance.* https://www.nice.org.uk/guidance/cg192.

98 **those who do see their babies:** I have found no literature on the experiences and effect on the bereaved of seeing and holding early miscarriages.

100 **Ariel Levy wrote about:** Ariel Levy, *The Rules Do Not Apply* (New York: Random House, 2017), 151; 145.

102 **take photos for parents:** Gifts of Remembrance, http://giftsofremembrance.co.uk/.

102 **US photographer Todd Hochberg:** Todd Hochberg, "Moments Held—Photographing Perinatal Loss," *The Lancet* 377, no. 9774 (April 16, 2011): 1310–11.

103 financially able to commission portraits: Rosemary Mander and Rosalind K. Marshall, "An Historical Analysis of the Role of Paintings and Photographs in Comforting Bereaved Parents," *Midwifery* 19, no. 3 (September 2003): 230–42.

104 more than one needed: The Sands 2016 survey suggests 91 percent of sixty-nine respondents had access to a cold or cuddle cot on their maternity unit.

104 required to be legally registered: The Births and Deaths Registration Act 1953 (as amended). However, although acknowledged on a legal register, stillborn babies won't be then recorded on a UK or US census, while they have been in Australia since 2016. Had Rose shown signs of life, such as breathing—she would have been a neonatal death, just as a baby born after twenty-four weeks but who also showed signs of life would too.

104 a miscarriage can happen: It's not quite as simple as this. In the US, there are state variations and eight definitions by combinations of gestational age and weight, although federal guidelines recommend reporting fetal deaths of 350 grams birthweight or twenty completed weeks' gestation if the weight is unknown. The definition of stillbirth in Australia is the birth of a baby who shows no signs of life after a pregnancy of at least twenty weeks' gestation or weighing 400 grams or more.

104 twenty-week boundary: R. H. Nguyen and A.J. Wilcox, "Terms in Reproductive and Perinatal Epidemiology: 2. Perinatal Terms," *Journal of Epidemiology & Community Health*, 59, no. 12 (2005): 1019–1021.

105 private member's bill: Civil Partnerships, Marriages and Deaths (Registration Etc.) Bill, https://services.parliament.uk/bills/2017-19/civilpartnerships marriagesanddeathsregistrationetc.html.

105 the issue of registration: *The Pregnancy Loss Review: Care and Support when Baby Loss Occurs Before 24 Weeks Gestation*, Department of Health & Social Care, March 2018, https://assets.publishing.service.gov.uk/government/up loads/system/uploads/attachment_data/file/693820/Pregnancy_Loss _Review_ToR_gov.uk.pdf.

105 conditions for its support: The Miscarriage Association, Position Statements, May 2018, https://www.miscarriageassociation.org.uk/about-us/the -charity/position-statements/.

107 sum up a fetal death: Fernanda Tavares Da Silva et al., "Stillbirth: Case Definition and Guidelines for Data Collection, Analysis, and Presentation of Maternal Immunization Safety Data," *Vaccine* 34, no. 49 (December 2016): 6057.

109 consent taking in this context: Miscarriage, Ectopic Pregnancy and Molar Pregnancy Bereavement Care Pathway p.10. Accessible http://www.nbcpath way.org.uk.

109 one perinatal pathologist interviewed: https://www.rememberingbaby .co.uk/. This quote comes from a video interview played at the exhibition.

112 a father's experience of stillbirth: Marcus B. Weaver-Hightower, "Waltzing Matilda: An Autoethnography of a Father's Stillbirth," *Journal of Contemporary Ethnography* 41, no. 4 (2012): 462–91.

114 Donating milk after pregnancy loss: In the piloting National Bereavement Care Pathway.

114 regulated human milk banks: UKAMB, Find a Milk Bank, http://www.ukamb.org/milk-banks/.

114 policies around donation: The Human Milk Banking Association of North America, Find a Milk Bank, https://www.hmbana.org/locations.

114 A newspaper in Philadelphia: Amy Wright Glenn, "On Gratitude and Grief: Mother Donates 92 Gallons of Breast Milk Following Pregnancy Loss," *Philly Voice*, November 25, 2015, http://www.phillyvoice.com/gratitude-and-grief-mother-donates-breast-milk-following-pregnancy-loss/.

Chapter Four: Again and Again and Again

120 the European Society of Human Reproduction and Embryology: Please see note 28 Chapter Two.

120 American Society for Reproductive Medicine: American Society for Reproductive Medicine, "What Is Recurrent Pregnancy Loss?," revised 2016, https://www.reproductivefacts.org/news-and-publications/patient-fact-sheets-and-booklets/documents/fact-sheets-and-info-booklets/what-is-recurrent-pregnancy-loss-rpl/?_ga=2.155439551.581550899.15315575 85-1901279129.1531557585.

121 set apart from the one-off: Raj Rai and Lesley Regan, "Recurrent Miscarriage," *The Lancet* 368, no. 9535 (August 12, 2006): 601–11. It is thought that 5 percent of women experience two consecutive miscarriages.

121 It is statistically rare: Henrietta Ockhuijsen et al., "Coping After Recurrent Miscarriage: Uncertainty and Bracing for the Worst," *Journal of Family Planning and Reproductive Health Care* 39, no. 4 (January 2013): 250–6.

121 often this cause is elusive: D. Ware Branch and Cara Heuser, "Recurrent Miscarriage," in *Reproductive Endocrinology and Infertility: Integrating Modern Clinical and Laboratory Practice,* eds. Douglas T. Carrell and C. Matthew Peterson (New York: Springer, 2010): 281–96.

121 one-third of women referred: Astrid M. Kolte et al., "Depression and Emotional Stress Is Highly Prevalent among Women with Recurrent Pregnancy Loss," *Human Reproduction* 30, no. 4 (February 2015): 777–82.

125 think more deeply about the language: The Miscarriage Association, "Films & Good Practice Guides," https://www.miscarriageassociation.org.uk/information/for-health-professionals/films-and-good-practice-guides/.

125 One guesstimate by a doctor: The Association of Early Pregnancy Units, http://www.aepu.org.uk/.

128 Words can shackle us all: Friedrich Nietzsche, *The Will to Power*, ed. and trans. R. Kevin Hill, trans. Michael A. Scarpitti (Penguin, 2017).

129 received medical wisdom: The World Health Organization suggested waiting six months, although anecdotally I often heard doctors advise couples to wait three months.

129 pregnancies conceived in the first: Chrishny Kangatharan, Saffi Labram, and Sohinee Bhattacharya, "Interpregnancy Interval Following Miscarriage and Adverse Pregnancy Outcomes: Systematic Review and Meta-Analysis," *Human Reproduction Update* 23, no. 2 (November 2016): 221–31.

130 in the context of waiting: As discussed in Sarah Bailey et al., "A Feasibility Study for a Randomized Controlled Trial of the Positive Reappraisal Coping Intervention, a Novel Supportive Technique for Recurrent Miscarriage," *BMJ Open* 5, no. 4 (April 2015): e007322.

131 conscious desire to hold back: Pegah Mehran et al., "History of Perinatal Loss and Maternal-Fetal Attachment Behaviors," *Women and Birth* 26, no. 3 (May 2013): 185–89.

131 defied her own usual rationality: Etsy, LoveYourBellyBelts shop, https://www.etsy.com/listing/229233999/fertility-belt-for-reproductive-health.

132 a plaster made from turpentine: Jennifer Evans and Sara Read, "'before midnight she had miscarried': Women, Men, and Miscarriage in Early Modern England," *Journal of Family History* 40, no. 1 (January 2015): 3–23.

132 idea of maternal impressions: Margrit Shildrick, "Maternal Imagination: Reconceiving First Impressions," *Rethinking History* 4, no. 3 (2000): 243–60.

133 simple means of support: Bailey, "A Feasibility Study." See note for page 130 above.

134 reminding of her life outside: This research supports the view that coping during RM may be eased by investing in as many aspects of life as possible. Paula L. Magee et al., "Psychological Distress in Recurrent Miscarriage: The Role of Prospective Thinking and Role and Goal Investment," *Journal of Reproductive and Infant Psychology* 21, no. 1 (2003): 35–47.

135 in 1800 43 percent of: Max Roser, "Child Mortality," *Our World in Data,* posted 2018, https://ourworldindata.org/child-mortality/.

136 "such ephemeral creatures as infants": Lawrence Stone, *The Family, Sex and Marriage: In England 1500–1800* (New York: Harper & Row, 1977), 651–2.

136 psychiatrist Colin Murray Parkes: Colin Murray Parkes, "Grief: Lessons from the Past, Visions for the Future," *Death Studies* 26, no. 5 (2002): 367–85.

136 similar indifference to miscarriage: Raymond A. Anselment, *The Realms of Apollo: Literature and Healing in Seventeenth-Century England* (Newark: University of Delaware Press, 1995), 59: discussing the entries of Elizabeth Freke, 1671–1714.

137 "the prism of miscarriage": Linda A. Pollock, "Embarking on a Rough Passage: The Experience of Pregnancy in Early-Modern Society," in *Women as Mothers in Pre-Industrial England: Essays in Memory of Dorothy McLaren*, ed. Valerie A. Fildes (London: Routledge, 1990), 39–67.

139 "non-mothering woman": Adrienne Rich, "Motherhood in Bondage," in *On Lies, Secrets, and Silence: Selected Prose 1966–1978* (London: W. W. Norton & Company, 1979), 195–7.

139 "constructions of normal femininity": Jane Maree Maher and Lise Saugeres, "To Be or Not to Be a Mother? Women Negotiating Cultural Representations of Mothering," *Journal of Sociology* 43, no. 1 (March 2007): 5–21.

140 scores of recorded insults: "The 10 Most Publicised Abusive Comments About Julia Gillard," *Tim Hein* (blog), May 22, 2012, https://timhein.com .au/2012/05/22/the-top-10-most-publicised-abusive-comments -about-julia-gillard/.

142 Erik Erikson, a developmental psychologist: Erik H. Erikson, *Childhood and Society*, 2nd ed. (New York: W. W. Norton & Company, 1963), 370.

143 "products" from their wombs: Shannon K. Withycombe, "From Women's Expectations to Scientific Specimens: The Fate of Miscarriage Materials in Nineteenth-Century America," *Social History of Medicine* 28, no. 2 (May 1, 2015): 245–62.

145 "at their lowest ebb": Andrew Moscrop, "'Miscarriage or Abortion?' Understanding the Medical Language of Pregnancy Loss in Britain; A Historical Perspective," *Medical Humanities* 39, no. 2 (2013): 98–104.

145 Those who preferred "spontaneous abortion": E. G. Clement et al., "The Language of Pregnancy Demise: Patient-Reported Clarity and Preferences," *Contraception* 96, no. 4 (October 2017): 300.

145 One researcher consciously writes: Paulina Van, "Conversations, Coping, & Connectedness: A Qualitative Study of Women Who Have Experienced Involuntary Pregnancy Loss," *OMEGA—Journal of Death and Dying* 65, no. 1 (August 2012): 71–85.

145 many feel that "loss": My thanks to Ruth Bender Atik for this crucial observation.

146 the physician Dr. Johann Storch: Barbara Duden, *The Woman Beneath the Skin: A Doctor's Patients in Eighteenth-Century Germany,* trans. Thomas Dunlap (Cambridge: Harvard University Press, 1998).

148 the effects of repeated miscarriages: Olga B. A. van den Akker, "The Psychological and Social Consequences of Miscarriage," *Expert Review of Obstetrics & Gynecology* 6, no. 3 (2011): 295–304.

148 remains epistemologically immature: Kimberly Fenstermacher and Judith E. Hupcey, "Perinatal Bereavement: A Principle-Based Concept Analysis," *Journal of Advanced Nursing* 69, no. 11 (November 2013): 2389–2400.

149 acute phase of grief: Norman Brier, "Grief Following Miscarriage: A Comprehensive Review of the Literature," *Journal of Women's Health* 17, no. 3 (April 2008): 451–64.

149 significant proportion of women: As quoted in Jessica Farren et al., "Post-Traumatic Stress, Anxiety and Depression Following Miscarriage or Ectopic Pregnancy: A Prospective Cohort Study," *BMJ Open* 6, no. 11 (2011): e011864.

150 **increase in stress and depression:** Astrid M. Kolte et al., "Depression and Emotional Stress Is Highly Prevalent among Women with Recurrent Pregnancy Loss," *Human Reproduction* 30, no. 4 (February 2015): 777–82.

150 **post-traumatic stress disorder:** Also see: Iris M. Engelhard, Marcel A. van den Hout, and Arnoud Arntz, "Posttraumatic Stress Disorder After Pregnancy Loss," *General Hospital Psychiatry* 23, no. 2 (March 2001): 62–6.

153 **how Tamang women speak:** Kathryn S. March, "Children, Childbearing, and Mothering," *Himalaya, the Journal of the Association for Nepal and Himalayan Studies* 10, no. 1 (1990): 6.

156 **she preferred to work alone:** Linda L. Layne, *Motherhood Lost: A Feminist Account of Pregnancy Loss in America* (London: Routledge, 2003), 48.

156 **or a woman's blood-clotting condition:** R. Rai and L. Regan, "Recurrent Miscarriage," *The Lancet* 368, no. 9535 (2006): 601–1. It is thought that 5% of women experience two consecutive miscarriages.

157 **or thrombophilia:** E.C. Larsen, et al., "New insights into mechanisms behind miscarriage." *BMC Medicine* 11, no.1 (2013): 154.

159 **reduce the chance:** Babill Stray-Pedersen and Sverre Stray-Pedersen, "Etiologic Factors and Subsequent Reproductive Performance in 195 Couples with a Prior History of Habitual Abortion," *American Journal of Obstetrics & Gynecology* 148, no. 2 (January 1984):140–6; H. S. Liddell, N. S. Pattison, and A. Zanderigo, "Recurrent Miscarriage-Outcome After Supportive Care in Early Pregnancy," *Australian and New Zealand Journal of Obstetrics and Gynaecology* 31, no. 4 (1991): 320–2.

159 **both time-consuming and expensive:** K. Clifford, R. Rai, and L. Regan, "Future Pregnancy Outcome in Unexplained Recurrent First Trimester Miscarriage," *Human Reproduction* 12, no. 2 (1997): 387–9.

159 **treating a patient's emotional world:** *The Investigation and Treatment of Couples with Recurrent First-Trimester and Second-Trimester Miscarriage*, Greentop Guideline No. 17 (April 2011): 13.

160 **supportive care in an RM clinic:** Anna M. Musters et al., "Supportive Care for Women with Recurrent Miscarriage: A Survey to Quantify Women's Preferences," *Human Reproduction* 28, no. 2 (August 2011): 398–405.

161 **the mourning behaviors of elephants:** Jeffrey Moussaieff Masson and Susan McCarthy, *When Elephants Weep: The Emotional Lives of Animals* (New York: Dell Publishing, 1995), 78, quoted in Deborah Davidson and Helena Stahls, "Maternal Grief: Creating an Environment for Dialogue," *Journal of the Motherhood Initiative for Research and Community Involvement* 1, no. 2 (2010).

Chapter Five: Ripples

165 **many men do the same:** John E. Puddifoot and Martin P. Johnson, "The Legitimacy of Grieving: The Partner's Experience at Miscarriage," *Social Science & Medicine* 45, no. 6 (September 1997): 837–45; Bernadette Susan McCreight, "A Grief Ignored: Narratives of Pregnancy Loss From a Male

Perspective," *Sociology of Health & Illness* 26, no. 3 (2004): 326–50; "Partners Too" survey http://www.ucl.ac.uk/news/news-articles/0714/21072014 -partners-of-miscarriage-sufferers-ignored.

166 **"only observes it":** Jon Cohen, *Coming to Term: Uncovering the Truth About Miscarriage* (Rutgers University Press, 2007), 9.

169 **number of men:** Anna J. Machin, "Mind the Gap: The Expectation and Reality of Involved Fatherhood," *Fathering* 13, no. 1 (May 2015): 36.

169 **a fourfold increase from 1989:** Gretchen Livingston, "Growing Number of Dads Home with the Kids," Pew Research Center, June 5, 2014, http:// www.pewsocialtrends.org/2014/06/05/growing-number-of-dads -home-with-the-kids/.

170 **secondary parent or support partner:** Machin, "Mind the Gap," 36.

170 **parental leave entitlements:** Mark Rice-Oxley, "MPs Call for 12 Weeks of Paternity Leave to Address Gender Pay Gap," *The Guardian*, March 19, 2018, https://www.theguardian.com/money/2018/mar/20/mps-call-for-12 -weeks-of-paternity-leave-to-address-gender-pay-gap.

170 **men are also far less likely:** "Survey of People with Lived Experience of Mental Health Problems Reveals Men Less Likely to Seek Medical Support," Mental Health Foundation, November 6, 2016, https://www.mental health.org.uk/news/survey-people-lived-experience-mental-health-prob lems-reveals-men-less-likely-seek-medical.

170 **Men can underestimate:** Omar Yousaf, Elizabeth A. Grunfeld, and Myra S. Hunter, "A Systematic Review of the Factors Associated with Delays in Medical and Psychological Help-Seeking among Men," *Health Psychology Review* 9, no. 2 (2015): 264–76.

170 **the annual Movember event:** https://uk.movember.com/?home.

173 **treatment of families in hospitals:** Hugh Jolly, "Family Reactions to Stillbirth," *Proceedings of the Royal Society of Medicine* 69, no. 11 (November 1976): 835–7.

174 **didn't forget the experience of miscarriage:** Until 1992, the legal cutoff for miscarriage was twenty-eight weeks.

174 **men can bond with their baby:** Hedwig J. A. van Bakel et al., "Pictorial Representation of Attachment: Measuring the Parent-Fetus Relationship in Expectant Mothers and Fathers," *BMC Pregnancy and Childbirth* 13, no. 1 (2013): 138; Anna R. Brandon et al., "A History of the Theory of Prenatal Attachment," *Journal of Prenatal & Perinatal Psychology & Health* 23, no. 4 (2009): 201.

175 **the Who's Your Daddy app:** http://www.whosyourdaddyapp.com/.

177 **similarly anxious husbands:** Jennifer Evans and Sara Read, "'before midnight she had miscarried': Women, Men, and Miscarriage in Early Modern England," *Journal of Family History* 40, no. 1 (January 2015): 3–23.

178 **It is the greatest griefe:** Ibid.

180 **male response to miscarriage:** Bernadette Susan McCreight, "A Grief Ignored: Narratives of Pregnancy Loss From a Male Perspective," *Sociology of Health & Illness* 26, no. 3 (2004): 326–50.

180 grieving in loosely binary ways: Terry L. Martin and Kenneth J. Doka, *Men Don't Cry . . . Women Do: Transcending Gender Stereotypes of Grief* (Philadelphia: Brunner/Mazel, 2000).

181 strength of the grief and anger: Gail Holst-Warhaft, *Dangerous Voices: Women's Laments and Greek Literature* (London: Routledge, 2002).

181 wailing songs of grief: Contact the Irish Traditional Music Archive in Dublin for more (https://www.itma.ie).

182 a male phenomenon in our consulting rooms: I have a well-received book on my consulting room shelf that also supports our experience: Alon Gratch, *If Men Could Talk: Translating the Secret Language of Men* (Boston: Little, Brown and Company, 2001).

184 male reproductive narratives: A recent study also shows how sperm counts have dipped enormously: Hagai Levine et al., "Temporal Trends in Sperm Count: A Systematic Review and Meta-Regression Analysis," *Human Reproduction Update* 23, no. 6 (November 2017):646–59.

184 less emotionally vulnerable: Quoting Cynthia Daniels's (2006) *Exposing Men: The Science and Politics of Male Reproduction* in Maria Lohan, "Advancing Research on Men and Reproduction," *International Journal of Men's Health* 14, no. 3 (2015): 214.

185 "My mates would only laugh . . .": Puddifoot and Johnson, "The Legitimacy of Grieving," 839.

185 fellow male bereaved: Daddys With Angels is one example of male support in grief after the loss of a child or in pregnancy: https://www.daddyswithan gels.org/.

187 We don't know why: Arthur Brennan et al., "A Critical Review of the Couvade Syndrome: The Pregnant Male," *Journal of Reproductive and Infant Psychology* 25, no. 3 (2007): 173–89.

187 men experience couvade: Maria Kazmierczak et al., "Couvade Syndrome Among Polish Expectant Fathers," *Medical Science Monitor* 19 (2013): 132.

187 teases a man for being "wimpy": Jenny Francis, "I'm Pregnant . . . and So's My Boyfriend," *The Sun*, updated April 6, 2016, https://www.thesun.co.uk /archives/news/890314/im-pregnant-and-sos-my-boyfriend/.

188 interior of the woman's body: Jan Draper, "'It was a real good show': The Ultrasound Scan, Fathers and the Power of Visual Knowledge," *Sociology of Health & Illness* 24, no. 6 (November 2002): 771–95.

188 men can feel excluded: Louis Locock and Jo Alexander, "'Just a Bystander'? Men's Place in the Process of Fetal Screening and Diagnosis," *Social Science & Medicine* 62, no. 6 (March 2006): 1349–59.

189 "stuck hot pokers": Puddifoot and Johnson, "The Legitimacy of Grieving," 839.

191 kept their feelings hidden: "Partners of Miscarriage Sufferers 'Ignored,'" UCL website, July 21, 2014, http://www.ucl.ac.uk/news/news-articles/0714 /21072014-partners-of-miscarriage-sufferers-ignored.

192 different ways of handling their grief: Of course there may be men who react genuinely unpleasantly. After Queen Katherine miscarried in 1514, Henry VIII was overheard cruelly taunting and reproaching her: John Guy, *Henry VIII: The Quest for Fame*, Penguin Monarchs series (Penguin UK, 2014).

193 higher risk of dissolving: Katherine J. Gold, Ananda Sen, and Rodney A. Hayward, "Marriage and Cohabitation Outcomes After Pregnancy Loss," *Pediatrics* 125, no. 5 (May 2010): e1202–7.

195 Turning to a mother: Paula Gerber-Epstein, Ronit D. Leichtentritt, and Yael Benyamini, "The Experience of Miscarriage in First Pregnancy: The Women's Voices," *Death Studies* 33, no. 1 (February 2009): 1–29. This paper is important for being one of the first studies published that explored in-depth the miscarriage experience, and here women talk about turning to their mothers.

199 sibling's experience of a late miscarriage: John P. Rosenberg, "'You Can Name Her': Ritualised Grieving by an Australian Woman for Her Stillborn Twin," *Health Sociology Review* 21, no. 4 (2012): 406–12. In Australia, "stillbirth" begins at twenty weeks.

201 "ghost" sibling acknowledged: Marcella Cameron Meyer and Steve Carlton-Ford, "'There but Not There': Imagined Bonds with Siblings Never Known," *Death Studies* 41, no. 7 (2017): 416–26.

202 "something to puzzle over": D. Rowe, *My Dearest Enemy, My Dangerous Friend: Making and Breaking Sibling Bonds* (Routledge, 2012), p184.

Chapter Six: Efforts to Remember, Pressure to Forget

206 early miscarriages happen at home: At least three UK hospital trusts recommend to miscarrying women in their patient information leaflets to flush their miscarriage away, as quoted in Sheelagh McGuinness and Karolina Kuberska, *Report to the Human Tissue Authority on Disposal of Pregnancy Remains (Less Than 24 Weeks' Gestational Stage),* (2017): 16, https://deathbeforebirth project.org/research/htareport2017/.

207 "People are horrified": Hadley Freeman, "Women Aren't Meant to Talk About Miscarriage. But I've Never Been Able to Keep a Secret," *The Guardian,* May 13, 2017, https://www.theguardian.com/lifeandstyle/2017 /may/13/hadley-freeman-miscarriage-silence-around-it.

208 one definition for ritual: Tatjana Schnell, "A Framework for the Study of Implicit Religion: The Psychological Theory of Implicit Religiosity," *Implicit Religion* 6, nos. 2 and 3 (2003): 86–104.

209 far from a modern practice: Vicki Lensing, "Grief Support: The Role of Funeral Service," *Journal of Loss &Trauma* 6, no.1 (2001): 45–63.

210 marking a profound transition: Corina Sas and Alina Coman, "Designing Personal Grief Rituals: An Analysis of Symbolic Objects and Actions," *Death Studies* 40, no. 9 (2017): 558–69.

210 **An ambiguous loss:** Paulina E. Boss, "The Trauma and Complicated Grief of Ambiguous Loss," *Pastoral Psychology* 59, no. 2 (April 2010): 137–45.

211 **deprived entry to heaven:** However, the International Theological Commission in 2007 assured parents of unbaptized babies that hope for their child's redemption isn't lost: "The Hope of Salvation for Infants Who Die Without Being Baptized," http://www.vatican.va/roman_curia/congrega tions/cfaith/cti_documents/rc_con_cfaith_doc_20070419_un-baptised -infants_en.html.

211 **Catholic rituals and symbols:** Maureen L. Walsh, "Emerging Trends in Pregnancy-Loss Memorialization in American Catholicism," *Horizons* 44, no. 2 (December 2017): 369–98.

211 **resources that guide ceremonies:** "Marking Your Loss," Miscarriage Association, https://www.miscarriageassociation.org.uk/your-feelings/marking -your-loss/.

212 **"fallen away from the church":** Lizzie Lowry, "A Letter to the Churches," *Saltwater and Honey* (blog), November 4, 2017, http://saltwaterandhoney .org/blog/a-letter-to-the-churches.

212 **A progressive rabbi:** Deborah J. Brin, "The Use of Rituals in Grieving for a Miscarriage or Stillbirth," *Women & Therapy* 27, no. 3-4 (2004): 123–32.

213 **tangible connections can help:** Inese Wheeler, "The Role of Linking Objects in Parental Bereavement," *OMEGA—Journal of Death and Dying* 38, no. 4 (1999): 289–96.

214 **they also supply boxes:** See: "Special Memory Boxes Set to Ease Grief of an Early Pregnancy Loss," NHS: Hull and East Yorkshire Hospitals website, https://www.hey.nhs.uk/news/2016/12/06/special-memory-boxes -set-ease-grief-early-pregnancy-loss/.

214 **three-sized boxes:** "Memory Boxes," SiMBA website, https://www.sim bacharity.org.uk/what-we-do/memory-boxes/.

216 **beautiful poem "Gift Wrapped":** My thanks to Clare Archibald for allowing me to use her poem. It was written for *Project AfterBirth* at the White Moose Gallery, https://www.whitemoose.co.uk/project-afterbirth -projects.

217 **manufacture of keepsake jewelry:** Lisa Mayoh, "Couples Are Turning Extra IVF Embryos Into Jewellery," kidspot website, July 3, 2017, http:// www.kidspot.com.au/parenting/real-life/in-the-news/couples-are -turning-extra-ivf-embryos-into-jewellery.

218 **"an elongated moment":** Brin, "The Use of Rituals in Grieving for a Miscarriage or Stillbirth."

220 **sensitive disposal options:** Sheelagh McGuinness and Karolina Kuberska, *Report to the Human Tissue Authority on Disposal of Pregnancy Remains (Less Than 24 Weeks' Gestational Stage),* (2017): 16, https://deathbeforebirthproject.org /research/htareport2017/.

222 **"a fetus is entitled to respect":** *Review of the Guidance on the Research Use of Fetuses and Fetal Material* (London: Her Majesty's Stationery Office, 1989), 20.

222 **Despite supporting guidance:** *Code of Practice—The Removal, Storage and Disposal of Human Organs and Tissue*, Appendix B: Disposal Following Pregnancy Loss Before 24 Weeks' Gestation, Human Tissue Authority, Code 5 (July 2006), B5.

222 **published around the time:** *Sensitive Disposal of All Fetal Remains: Guidance for Nurses and Midwives* (London: Royal College of Nursing, 2007).

222 **burning fetal remains:** Exposed in the Channel 4 *Dispatches* "Amanda Holden: Exposing Hospital Heartache," March 2014.

223 **guidance to the Scottish NHS:** https://www.sehd.scot.nhs.uk/cmo/CMO (2012)07.pdf.

225 **management of these gardens:** Kate Woodthorpe, *Baby Gardens: A Privilege or Predicament?* eds. Sarah Earle, Carol Komaromy, and Linda Layne (Farnham: Ashgate, 2012), 143-54.

227 **"I picked up the bag":** Hadley Freeman, "Women Aren't Meant to Talk About Miscarriage. But I've Never Been Able to Keep a Secret," *The Guardian*, May 13, 2017, https://www.theguardian.com/lifeandstyle/2017/may/13/hadley-freeman-miscarriage-silence-around-it.

227 **The most recent guidance:** *The Sensitive Disposal of Fetal Remains: Policy and Guidance for Burial and Cremation Authorities and Companies*, (London: Institute of Cemetery & Crematorium Management, 2015).

232 **to reveal its virtual inscription:** This message was accessed on July 11, 2017.

232 **chapter in the history of mourning:** Tony Walter, "New Mourners, Old Mourners: Online Memorial Culture as a Chapter in the History of Mourning," *New Review of Hypermedia and Multimedia* 21, no. 1–2 (2015): 10–24.

234 **Tommy's online "Book of misCOURAGE":** https://www.tommys.org/miscourage.

237 **Kahlo, who died childless:** Hayden Herrera, *Frida Kahlo: The Paintings* (London: Bloomsbury Publishing, 1993), 75.

237 **as described by the bereavement scholar:** Kenneth J. Doka, ed., *Disenfranchised Grief: Recognizing Hidden Sorrow* (Lexington, MA: Lexington Books, 1989), 187–98.

238 **many marginalized grievers:** Although there is a desperately moving video of fifteen-year-old Kirstie, uploaded to Facebook, about the late loss of her baby boy Jacob: https://www.miscarriageassociation.org.uk/story/kirsties-story/.

240 **launch of the first phase:** "National Bereavement Care Pathway to Be Piloted at 11 Sites," Sands website, August 1, 2017, https://www.uk-sands.org/about-sands/media-centre/news/2017/08/national-bereavement-care-pathway-be-piloted-11-sites.

241 **"you have already bonded with the bulge":** "Baby Loss Awareness Week," House of Commons Hansard, vol. 629, col. 267, October 10, 2017, http:// hansard.parliament.uk/commons/2017-10-10/debates/FF772C31-1540 -436B-BF50-8E4DD352458A/BabyLossAwarenessWeek.

Epilogue

252 **broad portfolio of research:** https://www.tommys.org/our-organisation /charity-research/miscarriage-research-centre.
253 **Miscarriage Priority Setting Partnership:** http://miscarriagepsp.org /introduction/.

Index